GET YOUR GLOW BACK AND RECLAIM YOUR ENERGY

DAILY REMINDERS TO INSPIRE HEALTHY LIVING

KATE TARRATT CROSS

© **Copyright 2022 - All rights reserved.**

The content contained within this book may not be reproduced, duplicated or transmitted without direct written permission from the author or the publisher.

Under no circumstances will any blame or legal responsibility be held against the publisher, or author, for any damages, reparation, or monetary loss due to the information contained within this book, either directly or indirectly.

Legal Notice:

This book is copyright protected. It is only for personal use. You cannot amend, distribute, sell, use, quote or paraphrase any part, or the content within this book, without the consent of the author or publisher.

Disclaimer Notice:

Please note the information contained within this document is for educational and entertainment purposes only. All effort has been executed to present accurate, up to date, reliable, complete information. No warranties of any kind are declared or implied. Readers acknowledge that the author is not engaged in the rendering of legal, financial, medical or professional advice. The content within this book has been derived from various sources. Please consult a licensed professional before attempting any techniques outlined in this book.

By reading this document, the reader agrees that under no circumstances is the author responsible for any losses, direct or indirect, that are incurred as a result of the use of the information contained within this document, including, but not limited to, errors, omissions, or inaccuracies.

CONTENTS

Introduction   v

Part I
WHAT TO KNOW SO YOU KNOW

1. DEFINE   3
   The Importance of Good Habits   5
   Flying With Habits   7

2. AND CONQUER   17
   The Game Plan   19

3. PUTTING IN THE WORK   33
   Setting Goals   34

   Flashcards and Templates   39

Part II
THE NUDGE

4. HERE COME THE WATERWORKS   47
   Why Water Gets the Job Done   49
   How Much Is Enough   53
   Jill's Troubles   58
   Get-Up-And-Go   58

5. COUNTING SHEEP   67
   What a Dream   68
   Problems With a 'Z'   75
   Where You Stand   77
   The Sleeping Pill   79
   Yawning Reflections   83

6. YOU ARE WHAT YOU EAT   87
   Let's Taco 'Bout It?   88
   Here Are the Harshmallows   91
   Eat Up! Wait... How Much of What?   92

Words of Encourage-Mints	93
A Real Pizza-Work	96

7. GYM AND TONIC 99
    Decisions, Decisions 100
    Active Habits 105
    Take It From Jeff 108
    Daily Dose of Iron 109

8. TAKING A STEP BACK 111
    What's the Priori-Tea 111
    Clearing the Way 114
    Yoga-na Do It 115
    Barking Rights 117
    Calming Chores 118

9. BREATHING 101 119
    Lung Lessons 120
    Keep Breathing 123
    Another One From My Library 124
    Wheezy Works 125

The Last Words 127
References 129
About the Author 143

INTRODUCTION

Even before I opened my eyes, I knew it was there. An extreme craving that tore me from my dreams. I turn onto my side and unlock my phone to look at the time. 4:15 a.m. It's really early. It's definitely too early for this. An acute hunger, unwarranted, yet dear to my heart. And they know it...

Salty, crisp lures, sitting in a dark corner, invoking me. I know they're there. Taunting me. They will stop at nothing to convince me, "It's not that bad!"—to get out of bed. Groaning, I try to convince myself to overlook them. *You're better than that. You're strong enough to shun them away. Ignore it, Kate. You can do it.*

Forget them...

I look up at the steady ticking clock on the kitchen wall, it's 4:25 a.m. It's early. With a loud rustle, the crimson bag clamps onto my fingers as it tries to stop me from pulling out its yellow innards.

Damn it! I did it again, haven't I? I've fallen right into their trap. But, I can explain. Really, I can. You see, I just... I couldn't resist. I just...

I just really love chips!

INTRODUCTION

I know what you're thinking, "You're a health coach! You should have things under control shouldn't you?" and all that stuff.

I know, I know, but look, I won't beat around the bush. Yes, I'm a health coach, and for the most part, I do have everything under control, it just so happens that I have a weakness for chips every now and then. But, you know what, don't we all have that one thing that buckles our knees?

I'm a human, you're a human, and we're all just humans trying to figure out what to do in the craziness that's our day-to-day. Thus, sometimes we do make mistakes and fall off the buggy, you know?

There's no point sitting around, moping about it. All there is to do is to be the change you want to see, to pull your socks up to your thighs, look on the bright side, say a couple more motivational sayings, and do what you have to do!

I've dedicated my life to helping nourish a variety of highly successful people by being the Masterchef of their dreams, not to toot my own horn, of course. I'm just joking around, but the point is that I've been around a lot of people, I've observed a lot of habits while learning and also learning about them for as long as I can remember.

With that said, I'm still your average Joe, and as you've come to know, I also fall off the wayside, but with my stern input about how habits could honestly shift your whole life, I'm on a trip to achieve bigger goals. That's why I'm here, to teach you what I know and walk along with you as you battle yourself to a better, healthier, and more successful future.

But, how Kate? How?! Well, the answer is as clear as day, as the answer is something we all know of, and probably also had at least once in our lives. I'm talking about straightforward habits!

Drinking water, sleeping, having good nourishment, being active, taking care of your mind, and just taking a breath.

I know by now you're probably reading this, deciding whether or not to continue with this read. I'm telling you that this isn't about some fad or trend that's popped up, this is about your health and happiness. This is about living a better life for you and your loved ones.

Remember that "All big things come from small beginnings" (James Clear, 2018). And your beginning is only starting now.

PART I

WHAT TO KNOW SO YOU KNOW

1

DEFINE

Habits are not a finish line to be crossed, they are a lifestyle to be lived.
–James Clear

Simply put, habits are little decisions and actions you make daily, which you do without lifting a finger or thought because when all is said and done, they become the norm.

Sounds pretty simple, right? I mean, brushing our teeth isn't a chore, is it? It's not something we think about. We just do it because it's what we need to do unless we want some missing chompers and people standing really-really far away!

We brush away because we were taught to do that from a very young age, and after continuously repeating this action, we made it a part of our day-to-day life. Even the ancient Chinese and Egyptians accepted cleaning their teeth as a health-must-do, although they used a lot more fish bones instead of brushes, and it involved tons of bark and sticks.

I'm getting carried away, of course. Habits aren't just about brushing your teeth and cleaning your pits. In truth, a significant sum of our everyday lives and our routines are made up of habits.

What would you say if I told you that habits account for about 40% of our behaviors on any given day? And this stat was only a fragment of the extensive research conducted at Duke University (Clear, 2018). Other breakdowns from neurobiologists, cognitive psychologists, and others argue that habits can even take up to 95% of our behaviors (Walesh, n.d.).

I know. It sounds kind of terrifying at first. We go about our days not realizing that half of our actions and decisions have been built into our brains. We're essentially striding around doing, thinking, and saying things without thinking about it because we've "gotten used" to doing it that way. I mean, talk about a lack of free will!

Well, back that up. It's important to understand that you're the only reason these "things" are duplicating. You did something, then you did it again, and again—up to the point where it became something you did all the time (and maybe forgot you were doing). So, forget about free will, you *are* in total control, and quite frankly, you've got all the power to shift, twist, and mold your habits, routines, and ultimately, your life. But, we'll get back to that later.

So, perhaps habits aren't as simple as we thought after all, right? Sure, the basic definition of the word "habits" can be put simply, but we could say the same about defining "flying," which would be something like moving through the air—for us humans, that's done with an aircraft (or witchcraft!). However, that doesn't help us understand what's going on in the cockpit, or prepare us for the inevitable intercom-ing *"ladies and gentlemen, this is your captain speaking."*

If we stick to the same image, habits are just like airplanes, really. The simplest form or definition would be analogous to the aircraft's shell. Then if you peek in a bit closer, you'll notice that there's a lot more to it: all sorts of sections, parts, and functions.

Keep in mind that I'm not trying to confuse or scare you away —I just find it cool to poke and pick at everything under the surface. By doing this, I hope to help you understand what habits are, how they fit in with your life, and how they outline who you are. From there on out, the chips will fall where they may, or in this case, the chips will fall where they are placed—by you… if that wasn't already clear enough.

So, in the next few pages, sit back, kick your feet up, and just relax while taking in some information, it will help lay all the groundwork to kick off your journey!

THE IMPORTANCE OF GOOD HABITS

Before we board for take-off, by now you're probably thinking, *Come on Kate, why should I care?! What have habits ever done for me?!*

Well, first off, calm down.

Habits are pretty nice to have around, and the good ones you've adopted have probably done a lot to push you through life without you even knowing it. With that said, if you think you're lacking a bit in the "healthy-habits" section these days, don't worry—that's why you're reading this in the first place, to improve and feel better about yourself. Good habits are very important but saying that doesn't mean a lot. You can't invest in a sales plan unless you get some more convincing, right? So here's the pitch!

A crucial reason that habits are so important is that they're like your "assistants," to push you through life and all the obstacles it throws your way. Like a glorious fleet of bulldozers, these assistants clear the path for you to reach for the stars and achieve your goals in life. Together, you become this unstoppable team! Although in actuality it's all you.

Ultimately, habits shape the foundation for your life. Think about it simply: If you were to run every morning or snack on healthier foods, you'll age much more gracefully because of your wholesome customs. You'll just live a healthier, better life in general, and who doesn't want that?

Drinking more water, exercising, sleeping better, and all those lettuce-like things are all ways your health will reap the rewards of your decisions. If I were to throw it in a list for you, it would look more or less like this:

- You could mold and maintain the body of your dream (or just a healthy weight will do).
- You'll have more energy to do other things you didn't have the time or strength for, ultimately increasing your overall productivity and charge.
- You'll get sick less, better maintain chronic illnesses (such as keeping your blood sugar in check), and you could possibly prevent ailments and diseases such as certain cancers.
- You'll have more control in your life, such as handling, kicking, and preventing toxic behaviors and relationships from slithering into your environment.
- You'll feel better in your own skin in terms of loving yourself and stepping up all of your *self's* like your self-control, self-esteem, self-confidence, self-respect, etc.

Embracing and caring for richer and healthier habits can shift your life into a whole other lane with changes and results that actually last in the long run. And that's another benefit of these healthy habits—their capability to outlast motivation.

Look, I'm not a fitness fanatic or gym buff, but when I first started working out, it was amazing! I would jump out of bed, fling on a jumpsuit, and just stretch and sweat! Then a week or two went by, and jumping out of bed became more of slinking out onto the floor and forcing myself to do a simple arm-lift.

Motivation is fantastic at first, but it doesn't last. However, when you force yourself to push past those dreadful days, you've got some new and improved habits on your hands! As for motivation? Forget about it!

If I were to "get real" with you about why it's essential to take that step and practice these habits again, well, it's simple: Everything listed and discussed above is taken from facts, information, and just a bunch of research. It's valid and genuine and all good. Clearly, the benefits are by the baskets, and you stand to gain a lot more than you would've if you were to press the skip button again.

Research aside, I can vouch for the change and necessity of "healthing-up" your lifestyle. You're here for a reason; don't deny or feel ashamed because you feel like you've fallen off the wagon, or even if you're only leaning off the side a bit, embrace, accept, and take that step!

You need these health-conscious yet austere habits in your life, such as clearing your mind and getting a good night's rest. You need to take care of yourself.

I know, I imagine you're all thinking, *But who has time for themselves these days?!* But look, what good does it do for anyone if your health is low-grade, you're all miserable and tired most of the time, and nothing's working out?! Here's some good ol' fashioned advice: Take care of *numero uno*, and everyone else will be just fine. Put yourself first, and what better way to do so than by doing a few simple things every day that you're not even thinking about! Remember that you're definitely not being selfish in any way. If you've been on a plane before, you probably know the oxygen mask speech that's coming. You're only human, and the human body and mind need their fuel and TLC to be the best they can be!

FLYING WITH HABITS

First and foremost, I would like to apologize sincerely to all the pilots and aircraft enthusiasts, especially those reading, out there. Let's clear the air: I'm neither of those. Airplanes are swell, but I'm no skipper or engineer. With that in mind, if I get some things wrong in terms of terminology or jargon, feel free to laugh it off and simply just enjoy the ride.

How Habits Form

We're skipping past the plane's body—or fuselage, wings, flaps, tail and all—to focus on the inside, and don't worry, you didn't take a wrong turn into a flight seminar. Just bear with me.

There are many sections within a plane, and probably one that is most well-known is the cockpit, which we'll use to show how habits are formed in our noggins.

A lot is going on inside the cockpit. A lot of buttons, pedals, and so on. However, I would like to focus on one specific thing called the *instrument panel*. If you drive, you'll probably already know what this panel is. If not, it's basically a panel that tells you all about the flight, engine, and everything meaningful for the pilots.

This information panel instantly made me think about our prefrontal cortex, which is a big chunk of the front of our brains responsible for decision-making. So, metaphorically, we've got this "panel" in our brains where information is displayed, like when we're trying to form new habits.

All habits start as a series of steps we take. It's like all the aisles and rows of seats on a plane which could be three steps or as many as 900 if you're more extreme. The point is that we decide to do steps one, two, and three. At first, these steps will require our time and concentration full-on as we're not used to doing these things. Then as time goes by and this series is repeated, the steps are moved to auto-pilot, meaning that there is little to no thought required to do them.

When the shift from full-on-focus to second nature occurs, the series of steps is lugged into a different part of our brains—the basal ganglia, a group of subcortical structures.

For this, we step outside of the cockpit, looking up at the overhead storage compartments.

The basal ganglia look like deflated oxygen masks and play a significant role in forming habits. Unlike our prefrontal cortex, the basal ganglia are free from the process of thinking and concentrate on the actions that lead to habit formation.

All of this might sound like a bunch of gibberish at first. The main thing to know here is that when we form habits, we acquire the pattern and repeat it to the point where it occurs automatically on cue or in certain situations. So, in the plane setting, the pilot will learn how to fly and fly a few dozen times while getting used to it until they sit in the seat and know what they're doing.

It's an entire process aimed to get the decisions and actions you make or those steps I was talking about locked up in your "storage compartment" or memory. Doing so will ensure that what you're flying towards becomes habitual and not something that's forced.

A Loop of Faith

I've found that a great way to demonstrate the basic framework of habits, and almost anything else, is to throw it together in some diagram or drawing. In this instance, we're lucky enough that Charles Duhigg already mapped out something called the Habit Loop. And yes, the loop is just how it sounds: a loop that holds the sway over any habit.

Of course, we have to stick with the image, so, as we know, planes have different travel classes, mainly first class, business class, and economy. Needless to say, you're business class, of course! However, as we're talking about the habit loop, we're not focusing on how much cha-ching you have, as habits don't cost a dime! Well, it depends. Still, we're only taking in some knowledge, and for this part, we're grouping the elements of the habit loop into these three classes.

Economy class: Cue (Trigger)

Business class: Routine

First class: Reward

Routine Airlines

I'm going to explain what each of these elements is. However, I will be jumping the loop and starting with the routine.

I saw this element and was like, "Oh, clearly, it's my day-to-day routine!" Well, not quite. Routine is the most apparent element when creating and reshaping habits because it's the habit itself. So, if you want to change a behavior, like giving up cigarettes, or reinforce some, such as drinking more water, then those things would be your routines.

Habit's routines are, for the most part, easy to identify. It's whatever you wish to change or reinforce. Since you were interested in reading this book, I presume that you wanted to change the way your day was steering by toughening simple habits, such as the way you eat. So, there you have it: your routine would either be one (or more) of the things we'll discuss later.

Also, note that there isn't an exact or "right" place to start, or else it wouldn't be a loop after all. However, I feel that this is the appropriate dropzone as we already know that our focus lies with simple habits. Yet, if later you find other habits you would like to tackle, simply follow the loop at first, and you'll find your way through it, seeing how and where you have to turn.

Once you've identified your routine, you'll have to do some further pinpointing for the cue and the reward.

Air Tri-Cue

Habitual cues or triggers are, simply put, things that make the habit happen. Our brains are great at making associations. When it comes to patterns, it's all the same. Our brains usually plant something to said habit, leaving behind a cue or trigger.

Before announcements, there are these *ding-dongs* on planes, and cues work the same way, more or less. When triggers jump up, internal chimes signal that something has to follow the tune.

Smokers' cues could be a cigarette with their morning coffee. Take a look at lunchtime. If you, for example, work next to a bakery or fast-food joint, you could get used to getting something quick to eat. Or, perhaps while changing your way of eating, the smell alone could trigger your brain to cue you in.

Nonetheless, these are your cues or examples of some, at least. Some people may consider some triggers to be more rugged than others. However, I don't think so. No matter how small the cue might seem, identifying them is relatively easy once you understand what they are. It's also necessary to do so as you're much more vulnerable in the early stages of changing, reinforcing, and making habits. The starting line of this process is where you'll have to put in a lot more effort to resist giving in to your cues.

A plane is a complex structure, and so are our brains. Our brains want the best for us, but sometimes it does more harm than good. Most of the time, our brains are on the chase to find pleasure. A part of our brain, the hippocampus, shaped like some of the earphones you get at the airport, is part of our internal reward system, and of course, we want some rewards!

Eating junk food, having lazy days, and staying up late, are things our brains hunt because it triggers our feel-good chemicals, such as dopamine. Thus, when we rob ourselves of experiencing these happy spikes, our brains get down. Nonetheless, it's only temporary. Our brains neglect and later lose these urges while replacing them with healthier resorts.

It's not rocket science, but, of course, nothing can be "just simple." Every time a trigger occurs before a habit, the linkage buffs up. Thus, the integration it has in our lives also strengthens, and a lot of the time, we're not even sure when the habit or trigger first occurred or how long it's been there. This makes it harder for us to break or replace old habits.

In short, your brain has created these connected channels and paths. So, if you were to roll a marble down it, it would follow down that specific route. Say you're on a flight that has reached quite a low altitude where you can see what's going on below you, and there's a canyon.

There will be all sorts of nooks, nicks, cuts, and crannies; some big, some small, some shallow, and some deep. Every time a habit is repeated with its trigger, the imprint will be etched deeper, making it more likely to happen again. The channel will also have more depth if the habit has been around for longer. Thus, as stated previously, more time and effort will have to be thrown into changing them.

Nonetheless, the way to change this would be to redirect the route up to the point where previous trails are neglected and later dumped altogether. Your way of thinking will reach some sort of default option, where you can then focus on carving out your simple habits.

Associating A (the trigger) with B (the habit) is about "neurons that fire together, wire together," as described in neuroscience (Sparks, 2021). Which is as accurate as it's catchy. This narrative stems from the Hebbian learning of Canadian psychologist Donald Hebb, which perfectly sums up the connectivity in everything we do.

The crucial thing to remember when not only identifying triggers but challenging them is to remember that whatever you do today will strengthen the chance of it happening tomorrow (Sparks, 2021). Therefore, shift your focus to better, healthier things now. Doing this means you'll be more likely to ignore bad habits and triggers while introducing newer ones easier in the future.

Having an understanding and knowing what our triggers are is essential. But, before I confuse us all, let's have a quick run-through of what these cues could look like in your everyday life. They're usually grouped together in two primary categories: internal and external cues, while a few subcategories fall under them.

The primary categories are exactly how they sound: internal cues being triggers that come internally, such as your mood, thought patterns, and other feelings, such as feeling tired. External cues come from the outside, such as your environment or location, people, places, and even the time.

In a later chapter, we'll jump in deeper regarding how we could utilize these factors to our advantage. However, for the sake of not piling on too much to remember, I think it would be best to move on to some rewards!

Rewards International

Rewards are simple. They're reasons our brains decide to stick to the steps we've taken. Why do we take flights? To get somewhere, to do something. We wouldn't just hop on a plane to nowhere without any reason, would we? We usually need something that makes the flight worth our time. Something has to drive us, right?

If we were to take simple habits, it could be anything from feeling "pumped" after a morning workout. Perhaps just feeling more energized and driven after having a good night's rest, or simply just enjoying some time to yourself while clearing your mind.

Rewards aren't always that easy to catch onto. Yet, as you experiment with different cues and routines, you'll find that one thing that drives your habits and your reasons for falling into them.

Let's say your focus lies with nourishment, and you've got a tendency to snack on chips or sweets when you get home from work. Not the best habit to have, but it happens to the best of us. Still, you want some change and healthier turn-tos. So, you decide to turn into bed early, but it doesn't seem to work as the fridge just keeps on calling your name! So, you try to drink some tea after dinner, or maybe you call up some friends to talk to until it's time to hit the hay.

Experimenting is key. Another key is to ask yourself if the reward you've now adopted is better than the reward you were settling for. Chocolate versus tea, socializing versus cheese puffs. Finding new ways to stimulate those feel-good chemicals is a great way to chase that extra *oomph* in your life. All while keeping things healthy. Just find a good way to keep a habit without feeling miserable and tired after trying to make it work. At first, it could feel like effort, but it shouldn't always feel like that. It should get easier and automatic as time goes on. If it doesn't, find something else to drive you so that it can come naturally.

On top of that, you'll possibly learn a lot more about yourself while doing this little experimentation, such as why you had certain bad habits; why you neglected some essential, straightforward ones; and where you have to go from there.

Habits clearly help us master the art of multitasking, as they're instinctive and require little focus and effort, allowing us to do more with our time. Turns out, they're a lot more complex than we could ever have thought, which is really cool if you think about it. There are endless opportunities and chances for you to take the plane by the nose and fly for air-you! I hope that's corny enough for you! If not, there's a lot more where that comes from, so stick around!

At the end of the day, the objective is to walk, or read out feeling greater and embracing the excellence that's you. I'm telling you, it's not now or never—it's now or now. So, all that's left to do here is turn the mirror to look after yourself and take care of yourself by reinforcing these simple and breezy habits.

However, what in the habit do you do now?! Where do you go from here? How does one quiet down the bad habits peeking under the covers, or where does one start with creating or reinforcing the habits we'll look at? Stress no more! As I've said, I'm right here as your habitual guide or whatever and all, so let's shimmy on over to the next chapter!

2

AND CONQUER

Old habits die hard, I guess. If you don't kick them, they kick you.
–Mel Gibson

There are two kinds of habits, and I'm sure you've heard me note it before, like some parakeet. Regardless, let me just run through it again quickly. Some habits are valuable in our lives and help us out in the long run, and then there are those which are the complete opposite. Good habits versus bad habits: the internal battle humans have been struggling with since days of yore.

As both of the determinants give away: good habits are good for us in the way that they're in a good shape to push us into the arms of our goals, whether it be your health, spending more time with your relatives, or simply focusing on finishing up on that book that's been gathering dust on your nightstand. Big or small, you can never have enough good habits.

With that said, and I think it goes without saying, bad habits are the ones we're worried about. They hold you back, push you away from your goals, and ultimately curb you from who you could be and what you can achieve. We can't imprint these simple habits without looking at which actions will stop them from being successful.

Let's look at some examples of bad habits we just can't seem to kick from time to time, which are also considered to be the top habits people struggle with these days (so, if you struggle with one or more of these, just know that you're not alone):

- We chomp down on junk food, fast-food, processed food, or sugary drinks (time to toss the crunchy papers, oily bags, and stomped-on cans!).
- We spend too much time on the phone or other electronics, such as social media or watching tv (we don't want square eyes, do we?).
- We have more lazy days than we like and neglect exercising (I know it's hard to pull on those running shoes sometimes, but we've got to try, right?!).
- We spend money on things we just don't need (Sometimes big spender, high roller, just leaves you at binge shopper).
- We take drugs or drink alcohol excessively (I'm going to have to step in as the fun police here, it's time!).
- We bag up the responsibility of others and neglect our own needs (which I know might not seem like a bad habit at first).
- We lose ourselves in our work and neglect our relationships (which is hard, we want to provide, but while the money comes in, you're losing more in the meantime).
- We do things like biting nails, picking our nose, or tugging at our hair (I can already hear my dad telling me to quit it).
- We smoke (whether it be cigarettes, vapes, or whatever else there is to smoke these days).

- We drink too much caffeine (which I only realized right now is a bad habit I would definitely have to kick... R.I.P.).

Once again, these are only a few habits that have popped on the radar. You know what you're struggling with and what the "habitual baggage" is you want to ditch. Maybe you have more than one habit you want to take on, or perhaps there are still some you're struggling to let go of. Wherever you stand, just breathe.

There is no right or wrong way when choosing the habits you want to leave behind, and I'm certainly not the one to tell you which ones you should strike! It's not my place, and nothing good comes from forcing someone to do something. I mean, it's like some people say, "Try telling a teenager to do something, and watch them do the opposite" —or something like that, I think!

We're all just overgrown children who can only transform and fully commit to change when it's on our terms. Sometimes, some of us just need that push in the right direction. That nudge to change your ways for the better!

So, the goal here is as clear as day: We need to break the bad and restock our lives with the good. Although we can't just jump on the horse wearing a blindfold—we need a plan!

THE GAME PLAN

The first step in changing bad habits would be to figure out why they're there in the first place. If you were to take an onion and look at its top layer, you'd find the most rudimentary and superficial marks; some would say that the bad habit's protective outer layer is boredom or stress—the thin shell of our true causes and problems. Some of us use boredom and anxiety to cover up our unhealthy patterns. All while ignoring what's really burning at the core.

You would much rather grab a drink on the weekend instead of sitting around doing nothing; biting your nails might just be something you've done to tone down the stress, and like, you've done it since you were a kid.

There are all sorts of core reasons we hold onto and jam into our internal jars of "things we do not speak about." Sometimes, we just don't like talking or thinking about certain things. *Bury and move on*; that's a motto many of us have accepted. We blame this, that, and everything that isn't "that thing." The explanation for this is simple; most of the time, we just don't like bringing up certain things as it's hard to do, we don't always know these things are there, and, you know, for the most part, it's just not fun to do.

I know that life gets busy sometimes and we get lost in all the responsibilities and challenges that it throws our way. That's life, and who are we to do anything about that? Regardless, we have *some* control over what we allow and turn down in our lives, and lucky for us, habits are one of them.

As briefly discussed in the previous chapter, there are several ways to catch/comprehend why we do what we do, such as looking at the rewards and triggers. I'll share a quick example of one method that sparked progress for numerous people I know (although it doesn't work for everyone).

They simply took an afternoon (some even took the day off to themselves), and they just sat. They started with a pen and paper or a screen and keyboard. Then they jotted down everything they could; mapping out, dot after dot, line after line. Scribbling and typing away, trying to find that *one core reason they allowed themselves to fall into these habits and why they haven't kicked them yet.*

It's all about asking yourself some hard questions, or simple ones that are tough to answer. You'll have to know who you are, and if not, take a deep dive into who that person is staring back at you in the mirror.

The process is formidable, especially for those who tend to lose themselves in life and what they're doing, those who don't focus on themselves, don't get any alone-time, and you know what… It will be hard. Few look at themselves from the outside perspective to judge and pick at all the things we do and where we took a wrong turn.

I mention this because there's one step in changing bad habits with the same building blocks as the exercise. The next part we'll be looking at, in my opinion, brings a lot to the table when it comes to turning things around.

Pulling the Trigger

We've learned quite a bit about habitual cues or triggers. When it comes to leaping past our bad habits and reestablishing simple ones in their place, identifying these "alarms" is the way to go!

The one and only great way to figure things out is to observe and record. Simple as that.

When you decide to tackle the game plan, you have to concentrate on what you're doing throughout your day, keeping an eye out for those habits you're trying to lose. Then when they stride along, grab your writing instrument of choice and see whether you can answer at least one of these questions:

- Where were you when the habit happened?
- At what time did it come along? (Could be specific, such as 2 p.m., or general, such as in the evening.)
- What were you feeling before it happened and when it happened? (It could be your mood, thought patterns, or other senses, like feeling sleepy or sick.)
- Were there any other people involved? Who were they?
- Did it happen right after something else? What was that something?

These might seem like dumb questions for identifying triggers, but things start clearing up once you read between the lines. Location, time, internal behaviors, people, preceding events. Sound familiar? These questions all include the internal and external cue categories we've talked about. Thus, these questions are the basic framework for mapping out where your triggers stand.

Picture this; *A person sits alone in an office all day performing various tedious tasks. After work, it's half an hour of stop-go traffic. Then at home, it's throwing together dinner, scrubbing and mopping a bit, taking care of the kids, getting everything ready for the next day, a shower, then bedtime.*

This is a very average routine. We're all just busy little worker ants, after all.

Back to the example: In between the very active schedule they have going on, this particular person drinks two to three energy drinks during the day and chows down on cookies and other snacks around the home while preparing dinner and packing lunches. They go to bed still soaked from the shower because clearing their mind or relaxing isn't on the to-do list, and they just want to sleep!

For this person, I would say that places, people, time, and preceding events don't play a leading role in their triggers (although they could). Internal cues are a definite factor: This person is clearly overworked with tasks, they're bored, frustrated, and lonely at work, and by the time they're at home, they're exhausted. This person tries to get some energy and drive with caffeinated drinks; they snack because they're most likely hungry and still have a lot to do at home, so eating a healthy dinner might seem like "more work" for them to do. They don't take time to themselves because they've overworked themselves to the point where they just want to sleep and put the day behind them.

This person's best shot at change would be to take a step back to look at their surroundings, triggers, and schedule. They're bored with their work, but so are many of us. However, the majority of us can't pack up our things and leave our day jobs. Although looking around for other job opportunities isn't the craziest thing to do. Just know that it's something that needs to be discussed and thought about thoroughly, not an impulsive act to try and force change. It's a risky chance to take, so don't jump to doing that right away unless absolutely necessary.

There are other ways to deal with your triggers and reinvent your life. For starters, this person can gain a lot from implementing some *time management* into their life. With the focus on habits and triggers alone, this person can also benefit enormously from *managing their emotional state* and responses to them while adding in alternatives. For example, when they feel bored and frustrated at work, they can turn to drinking water or tea instead of energy drinks. Perhaps they can replace the habit of drinking (not alcohol) with other things, such as a quick meditation at noon to pull themselves together and unwind. They could even, for example, try to make their dull tasks more fun by setting up goals and challenges for them to complete and being creative with the tasks before them.

There are endless routes to take once you've spotted your triggers. You could either eradicate the habit altogether or change the rotten routine—by either setting up new triggers, taking on new patterns or alternatives, and so much more.

The above example only scratched the surface of dealing with habits after you've identified triggers. All these cues (their categories) can look different in various lives.

Answering the questions from earlier is a great way to categorize your triggers. Placement alone, however, isn't enough to spark a difference. Knowing how to use them afterward is probably the most meaningful step. When we tap into the categories of triggers and how we could use them to our advantage, things really cock to the side and into a new perspective. So, let me stop rambling and give it to you straight!

Tapping Into Utilization

We'll run through this going from *a* to *b*, starting with preceding events.

Preceding events are, as previously characterized, the events that happened directly before a habit. These events form a part of our "habit structures" in the shape of trigger actions that push our daily routines to transpire. We can use these to our advantage when trying to implement new habits, such as stacking together habits with other automatic habits that are tied to one preceding event. Make sure that your event is something you will always do no matter what, like getting in and out of bed—this is a highly recommended timeframe to push your preceding events into, because your body is still low on energy. So, more automatically, your body will get used to these habits because your focus and fuel aren't invested in the events and the routines to follow.

You could say, for example, "When I get out of bed, I will drink a glass of water while taking my vitamins." Or, "Before I turn off the night lamp, I could take a minute or two to read a few pages of that dusty book" that I mentioned earlier.

Preceding events are all about knowing when to kick over the dominos of routines and habits. So that when they are in play, the motion means all of your habits are more likely to happen.

This brings me to time. I know they say it's money, but be genuine: Everything revolves around time. *How much time do I have to do this? When am I going there? How long is this?* Or, *That was quick!* Time rotates around us, all the "time." That's why time could be considered a valuable and powerful trigger choice: There's no leeway; time always happens, so it will be a recurring spur, which is a great way to ensure an action becomes a habit.

That said, I lose track of time all the time! Most of us don't have an internal clock on the wall, thus making us bad timekeepers. This could make us steer away from time triggers when, in truth, there's a simple way around our forgetfulness.

Most of us are blessed to have digital means to remind us of the time, such as alarms, app notifications, and scheduled events. These mentioned few are precisely how we could use time to help us create triggers and habits. Take out your phone, and set a recurring labeled alarm to do whatever it is you have to do once it goes off. Then with calendar events, you could add your weekly or monthly goals, and they will remind you when the time comes around. App notifications could work in the same way as the alarms. There are so many apps out there, one that's a "beer glass" and one that's "hand sanitizer" (I'm more than a little skeptical about that one), so I promise you that you'll find an app that fits with your goals and habits you want. Do you want to exercise more? Get an app that could remind you during the day to exercise or send you a message at a specific time you want to meditate. Remember the following; never dismiss an alarm for a habit that's not yet completed. Rather snooze than shirk.

The next factor you could pull into your life to keep you motivated to create and maintain habits is to take responsibility for your actions. Doing so could help you build and improve your relationships, as well. Not to sound in any way sinister or wicked, you can use other people as triggers for habits.

With Whom You Surround Yourself

There are two parts to "other people" triggers: The people you surround yourself with (the company you keep) and the people you pull along in your journey.

When it comes to the company you keep, I can sum it up with two quotes you might know, "You are the average of the five people you spend the most time with," from Jim Rohn (Motivation

Supply, n.d). "Be wary of the company you keep for they're a reflection of who you are, or who you want to be" (Ortiz, n.d.)

I've heard this my whole life, how it doesn't matter who you are if you associate yourself with the wrong people, you too will be viewed as they are. Now, I'm not hinting that you should open the door and start kicking everyone out one after the other. Unless someone is bad or toxic for you and your life, you don't have to be drastic. It's all about surrounding yourself with the people that want the best for you while spending less time with those who don't.

Friends often unconsciously encourage or vandalize behaviors they value and don't value, including some habits. Thus, when you're removing or creating them in your life, it's necessary to sit down and talk to the people in your life so that they can support you. However, you have to have *the talk* so that they can understand where you're coming from, what your motivations are, and how they can help you, such as calling you out when you dip off the wagon. Meet in the middle where needed, and communicate until you all are on the same page.

The second part is all about forming a small pack with family or friends that have the same goals as you. This way, you'll have someone who "understands what you're going through," and you could support one another and hold each other accountable.

The best way to utilize these "other people" triggers is to get your social mountings in place. Join communities and spend more time with people who have the same values as you, learn from them, and take the feedback, criticism, corrections, and advice others have to give.

You could also start grouping up with others, such as joining a yoga class. That way, you could be around others aiming for the same goals as you. Another great way to ensure that you go through with this trigger is to pre-commit to the plans you make, prepay for that yoga class, schedule with friends in advance, etc.

That leaves us with two categories of triggers to cover. The first one of the two will be your surroundings because you know that they say: location, location, location.

Think about all your surroundings, the places you go to (almost) every day: your home, office, perhaps the nearby supermarket. All, or most, of these places, have habits (good or bad) attached to them.

Perhaps you drink a lot when you're at home, overstress at work, hunger-shop at the supermarket. And vice versa with the good. Your best shot would be to overwrite these triggers, replacing them with things that help us reach our chosen habits.

There are a few ways you could go about this:

- Avoid locations that spring up bad habits (such as bars, fast-food joints, etc.). When it's impossible to do so (like in your home or office), you could remove the thing (usually physical) from that surrounding. So, for example, remove the alcohol or certain foods (temptations) from your home.
- When enforcing a good habit, ensure that the "tools" you need to complete it are set in your locations. Whenever the thing catches your eye, it will act as a reminder for you to complete the habit. You could also gain some motivation since there will be no more "where is it?!" and hunting down things anymore.
- You could also try breaking down sections of each location where you can. Let's say we're taking a tour of a home. There's a space for creative work, client-related work, relaxation, socialization, cooking/eating, and the rest. This apparent divide could help you use your location and environment for your own good. Let me explain. You've hit a roadblock with creating advertisements, so you go over to working with some

clients or take some time to relax. Then, when you're done, you get something to eat before dashing back over to the ads.

Location, at first glance, looks like a tough cookie to take on, but as you can see, it's not as tough as it seems. It's all about placing yourself in the proper space to achieve your habitual goals. As you've seen, there are ways around bad triggers that don't involve you ditching your job. All you have to do is recognize, eliminate, replace, and step out of your own way, and that goes for all the trigger categories!

Last but not least, we have emotional triggers. This one is, by far, the trigger category that's to blame for most of our bad habits and the one we most struggle with. The key to dealing with these triggers, such as being anxious or upset, is listening and owning them.

You're a person who has feelings, thoughts, and emotions—it's as normal as breathing. However, when we ignore these things and drown them out with something else, like food or Instagram, we allow bad habits to form and cloud our minds and judgment.

Therefore, there's only one thing you can do. You'll have to recognize what you're feeling. Are you feeling mad? Unhappy? Stressed? Whatever it may be, even if it's happy, identify what you're feeling, why you're feeling like that, what has caused it, and all that jazz.

Doing so allows you to slow down, take a breath, and figure things out, which ultimately means you have more control over what you'll do next and which habits you'll respond with. You could also try and "trick" these triggers by nestling small patterns (habits) to help you cope with negative emotions, feelings, and thoughts. This can be anything from journaling, listening to music, going for a run, and so on, but note how you could even eliminate these triggers by adding the simple habits straight on? This will help you have these healthy habits in the future, even when you're down in the dumps.

Up Next

When it comes to setting up a foolproof game plan, dealing with triggers is only one play of the book. However, I can already feel your eyes getting heavy, so this will be quick.

The first step to changing and making habits is the clearest one of them all, and that's to take a close look at yourself, your habits, and what you'll need to change things. I think I've mentioned and made this clear a few times, so that's all I'll say.

The next step or advice would be to start small. The tortoise called it, "Slow and steady wins the race!" He couldn't be more right! Squashing ourselves under multiple habits, goals, and things to do, doesn't help anyone, especially not you. You're only one person, so don't overdo it.

Start small, take on a single habit, or do one small thing to work towards a few of them. For example, take a jug of water to work, do 100 jumping jacks at home, and do one thing for yourself before bed. See what I mean? Even though you're concentrating on more than one habit, you're still keeping things light and steady so as not to overwhelm yourself. Remember, there's enough time to increase the speed and quantity at a later stage. Don't jump right in with a barrel of cheese on your back!

You should also be intentional when you pick your habits from the lineup. Prioritize them from the most influential in your life to the least. Also, be realistic and clever. Meaning: don't aim for a habit that impacts your life negatively, even if it's only for now.

So, for example, don't try to take on Ice Hockey if you know you can't afford it at the moment. There's always later, once you've tackled some other habits. It could also be something simpler, like selecting a skill learning course that works for your schedule and not one that will require you to shift your whole week, plans, and schedule.

Another thing, if you find that you're struggling with exercising, think to yourself if that's really the only thing you should be looking at. Balance is essential in life. Without it, you'll always be, well, unstable. As Jana Kingsford said, "Balance is not something you find. It's something you create." (Gill, n.d). This perfectly sums up what you should be running towards a healthy and happy life, balanced in all areas. By all areas of your life, I'm talking about the savory seven:

1. environment (everything around you, including your home, workspace, etc.)
2. career
3. finances
4. relationships
5. personal growth (your relationship with yourself and self-improvement)
6. mental health
7. physical health

If we look at our simple habits, our physical, mental, and personal growth goals will take the top spot. In most cases, your relationships, career, and environment will also benefit from these habits and lifestyle changes. But you'll find that out on your own.

The bigger picture here is to make sure all the areas of your life have at least one good habit. I know I said to start small, and as I've shown, it's still possible to take on more than one habit while pacing yourself accordingly.

However, not all of us want to focus on more than one habit at a time, which is just fine. Focus on one thing. You could always take on one, and then after you feel you've gotten used to it, you could take on the next one, and then the next one, until all the pieces are pushed together, and you've got the whole pie on the plate!

Then, most importantly, you have to celebrate every victory you make, no matter how little. Set up a system that allows you to grab onto a sense of triumph. It will help keep you motivated. And you could see and feel the progress you're making. Celebrate your wins, even if it's only remembering to drink one extra glass of water. It's the small stuff that adds up and counts in the end. You don't need a group of people standing in the same outfit with pom-poms shaking vigorously—be your own cheerleader! So remember to pat yourself on the back. Scream out, "Great job!" or "I'm amazing!" every now and then, and always keep habit-ing forward!

3

PUTTING IN THE WORK

You're always one decision away from a totally different life.
–Mark Batterson

When it comes to health and being healthy, it could look different and mean different things to everyone. Some might think that "health" means you're a total gym buff who only eats protein, while someone else might think that exercising a few days per week is well-over good while eating less restricted is the way to go. Health doesn't have to be yanked out from the dictionary to mean the same thing.

When answering the question below, be creative and honest with your approach. Remember. Don't just go with what you were taught, such as eating your fruits and veggies (although they really are healthy), running around, and being a size zero, is the way to go about health. Think about your answer. Take into perspective who you are, your priorities, goals, and what your life looks like, or more notably, what you want your life to look like. It could be anything from not waking up with no energy and drive for the day, spending more time with your children, or spending less time with them (for those parents who are allocated 0% privacy), eating more homemade meals, and making an effort to do simple things, such as caring for and creating habits, like those simple ones many of us forgot. So, answer me this:

What does health mean to you? (Give your general definition)

Great! Now see how many of the six simple habits you can spot in your answer.

SETTING GOALS

Before we can run, we have to stretch, so we can't jump over the definition of goals. I know most of us understand what goals mean and have probably clutched many of them. However, scribbling down a quick guess isn't enough to comprehend what goals mean in full.

Crash Course on Goals

"A goal is an idea of the future or desired result that a person or a group of people envision, plan, and commit to achieve." (Ho,

2020). I couldn't have defined it better myself! Which is why there are quotation marks…

Nevertheless, moving on. Habits and goals are very much the same in that they're both a lot more complex than they appear on the surface. Of course! And in all clearness, when creating and reinforcing habits, you'll have quite a lot to do with goals.

Goals contribute to our visions, dreams, and desires. People often confuse these, but they're different by a long shot. These things are simply the stepping stones we take to reach our goals.

There isn't just one goal type, though. You could, once again, cram different sorts of habits into different categories. However, they are usually either time-based or life-based, sometimes both.

With **time-based goals**, there are three categories we could look at: daily goals, short-term goals, and long-term goals.

Daily goals are those tiny tasks you can get done within a day. They often act as objectives for long-term goals and could also be recurring. *Short-term goals* go on for longer, such as a few days or a week, and they could also lend you a helping hand for long-term pursuits. Then there are *long-term goals*, which are more extended in outstretched periods. It can go for months, years, and sometimes even the majority of your life.

When we take a look at the simple habits, we can try to make it look like this, more or less:

- Daily goal: Running every morning.
- Short-term goal: Comfortably run 6 miles within a month.
- Long-term goal: Join a marathon, or maintain a cardio routine.

Then with **life-based goals**, there are career goals and personal goals.

Career goals are obviously related to your profession, while personal goals have everything to do with your personal life. *Personal goals* emphasize your health, so your happiness and composure as an individual. As well as most of the simple habits we'll look at and most of the goals we make in general.

We're most likely sticking with one long-term goal: getting healthy and keeping our simple habits in place.

You'll achieve this by breaking down this goal into smaller pieces to chew in the form of daily and short-term goals. Hold on now, don't just dive into the deep end! You have to play this smart, and the best way to do so is to set up SMART goals that are aligned with your life purpose and core values, prioritized to impact your life the most, and finished off with an action plan.

SMART goals are specific, measurable, attainable, relevant, and time-bound. These five factors are the ideal ingredients to ensure the perfect recipe for well-defined, detailed goals that aren't genetic or wide. Your goals should leave no wiggle room, and they should be realistic, or once again, they should be SMART.

They should also fit in with what you want to do and be in your life and core values. Then you should sit down by yourself and decide which goal is worth taking on first if it benefits you the most. The thing is, I can't tell you what you have to put first. No one can. Only you can decide and prioritize.

People often use vision boards to display and keep track of their goals. On these boards, you can go all out! You might stick on some photos of cars, a silhouette of a couple, or a rising chart for your career goals, etc. It can look like there are so many goals, and most of the time, there are a lot of photos and post-its, but that's where you have to narrow down on your vision, or else there would be too much to handle and you won't be able to focus on the right things.

Look, sign me up for a Lamborghini if you can, but if I know that my relationships need some work, I should definitely focus on those first. Like I said—slim down your focus on smaller, more important goals to help you become the best you can be while still keeping your loved ones in mind.

Then all that's left is to sketch out a plan of action. After all, setting up your goals isn't enough to get the ball rolling. You need an outline that breaks down your goals into smaller, more attainable milestones. The actions you take daily to make sure that your plans become reality.

When you look at goals and what you need to do to achieve them, doesn't it become clear that they are frankly habits that you work on regularly, or could be attained through daily habit changes? Yes, that was a rhetorical question because that's absolutely what habits and routines are: Small goals and small steps you take to make habits that stick around.

So, remember why you wanted to take on these simple habits again: Why did you pick this book from the lineup? What is driving you to live a better, healthier life? Hold onto that thought throughout (even when times get rough), because that's the only way you'll walk out with some sturdy habits on your hips.

FLASHCARDS AND TEMPLATES

What are your goals? (List them, but remember to do so using detail and SMART goal factors)

What are some steps you'll take to reach your goals?

Who could help you reach this goal? (Friends, family members, parents, support groups, etc.)

Are you assigning yourself specific deadlines for these goals? How much time did you give for each goal? Are they realistic and attainable?

What are your strengths and challenges? Are there any areas where you know you struggle with maybe? How will you address these concerns, and use these strengths to your advantage?

What are your action steps? Which action steps have you taken? Do you think some steps aren't working as you thought they would? How will you change, shape, and replace these steps?

(Once you've started) What did you find easy, and what did you find hard in picking out your goals and moving towards them?

Answer these questions every day (for the first one), every month (for the second one), and the third one every year. You could also change the last one as time goes on and your priorities shift.

I want this for tomorrow...

I want this for the end of the month...

I want this for the end of the year...

I want this for the end of my life...

Do you have any notes for yourself? Ideas, advice, criticism, encouragement, anything?

Or, take a moment and try to set up some SMART goals, focusing on the simple habits (where applicable) and concentrating on where you're lacking in your life.

1. Write out your goals (roughly is fine).
2. Then prioritize them in a top-five list (leaving the rest of them on another list).
3. Do your research on ways to achieve this goal and make notes on this.
4. Write out a detailed plan of action with some action steps to take, deadlines, progress bars, and whatever you feel can make your "program" more alluring and fun. All while keeping in mind everything you have to, facts and all, and remembering that you're talking about simple habits here. Even though you could use this chapter for other areas in your life. Still, try and see how you could add all of this together to help you push toward creating and strengthening simple habits.
5. You could also create something to motivate yourself to remember and stick to these habits, such as our old

friend the vision board, then there are also mind-mapping your goals, keeping a journal, using habit/goal trackers (applications), or you know, something as simple as telling a friend about your accomplishments.

PART II

THE NUDGE

4

HERE COME THE WATERWORKS

Pure water is the world's first and foremost medicine.
–Slovakian Proverb

As the late and great Mr. Bruce Lee said, "be water." Now, of course, he was being a lot more philosophical and "zen" when he had said this. The point is that when I say it to you, I'm talking about actual water. Still, *tomayto-tomahto, potayto-potahto*! The human body is, on average, made up of 60% of water (The USGS Water Science School, 2019). Thus, to stick with the whole zen feel, you are water, and water is you.

Nonetheless, Mr. Lee definitely had something going with his quote, so we might as well take a dive into it as there's a lot to learn from it. It might even leave you feeling more motivated to take on your goals for drinking water and the others to follow.

For those who don't know who Bruce Lee was, he stood as a martial arts luminary and later became an overall jack-of-all-trades. Lee was also a polymath who released a lot of inspiring quotes as he trained and learned the art of fighting. During his early years of training, Lee learned about the admirable qualities of water. He knew he couldn't strike water, no matter how hard and robust his punch was. Water was the opposite, being able to punch through very tough substances. Lee wanted to be just like water and did so (not literally) through the art of detachment, which is all about "detaching" yourself from reality by clearing your mind and relaxing.

You see, Lee admired the qualities of water and thought that we should all be like it, meaning that we should be without form. What he meant to say was that we shouldn't trap ourselves in a single mindset and always strive for growth and change. Water adapts to almost everything, becoming whatever we jam the liquid into water bottles, cups, or teapots. So, with that image in mind, Lee meant that we should also be able to "jam" ourselves into any situation and then acclimate, develop, and transform.

Nevertheless, here, to "be water" is more about drinking water. I know, what a disappointing turn of events (not really, though). Now, if your earlier independent life was anything like mine, you know how critical water is. I can't even begin to count how many times someone, be it my parents, doctors, or teachers, had told me to drink my H^2O, especially when it was hotter outside. Of course, back then, being a stubborn teenager was like, "Yeah, but I'd rather not," and then grabbed some soda on my way out. Yet, as time grew on me, I realized that I was wrong, they were right, and water is the most important meal of the day—well, the most important drink anyway.

Then again, drinking water is sometimes easier said than done. Many people firmly believe that water is (a) tasteless or (b) horrendous. On the contrary, I'm someone who enjoys the taste of water, especially after some hard work in the summer. So, we'll just have to agree to disagree. At least, if you're not a fan of water, there are some ways around that, which we'll go through later in this chapter.

Yet still, those of you who like water also face some challenges from time to time. Personally, I struggled with remembering to actually drink the water. I would literally have the bottle next to me and get so carried away with work that I only took a few sips here and there, and with those sips, I ended up drinking way too little. Many people have the same problems, either forgetting to drink their liquids, or drinking water but not enough—or in my case, both. Luckily, as I said, there are some ways around that too, but we'll get there when we get there.

What to take from all this playful wordiness is that water is essential to our bodies, and that we can't go without it. Just imagine what could happen if we were to take drinking water and thread it into our day-to-day as a habit.

WHY WATER GETS THE JOB DONE

I don't know about you, but I can't remember half of the things I've learned in school, especially if I wasn't interested or didn't enjoy the subject. For most people, that's biology. I get it. Sometimes, it can get draggy and boring. Today, however, we'll be getting a bit biological—not a lot, but enough.

Think of one of those posters in almost every doctor's office and seventh-grade science classroom: That one with the basic human frame and multicolored organs, all assigned with their fitted labels.

If I were standing there, swinging around one of those long silver pointer sticks (or more likely, a laser pointer), I would explain that when it comes to drinking water, we would start at the mouth—obviously. After we have flooded our cheeks with water and swallowed, the water travels down our esophagus, that tube connecting our throat and stomach. Like everything you swallow, good and bad, that's where the water ends up—in your gut.

The key difference between water and food within the stomach is that water isn't "digested" as food is. On the contrary, digestion is sped up by adding water to the menu. That's why most people suggest drinking water before, during, and after meals—it helps quicken up digestion and soaks up all the nutrients offered by food. It won't be "digested" or taken through the bowels as our food will, but rather the water is absorbed as it goes.

Water absorption starts in the stomach and then that sweet sweet H^2O is pumped into the bloodstream. While this is happening, water is also passed through the smaller intestines and further sponged into the blood.

From there, it's express galore. Water travels to cells all over the body. This hydration is why water is so significant to our bodies. So that our cells and organs, such as our kidneys, can do their best job. That brings me to another thing water helps with: filtration.

We have what are basically internal coffee machines, where things have to be filtered out into a "cup," or in this case, the bladder, for the most part. Kidneys are the sheriff in town when cleaning our systems from all tainted toxins. However, they require some energy to do so efficiently, that charge being water. Without this soggy fuel, our health is affected, causing kidney-related diseases such as kidney stones, which are most common.

Water also helps scrub away toxins from the skin, leaving your skin advertisement-like: hydrated, healthy, stretchy, and less wrinkly. Then at the end of the cycle, water comes out of the body when we sweat and visit the powder room.

I saved this part for last because it really stood out to me, and I don't know if many people know quite what influence water has on our brains.

When we drink water, our brain cells are hydrated, which means they can "grip on" more. Especially when it comes to our cerebral functions (all of our conscious mental activities, such as thinking, reasoning, moving, and talking). You'll also have this burst of cognitive performance, where you'll be able to process more information with better attention and concentration. All of which we need to start with our simple habits.

On top of that, our mental health will have some fixing, dusting, and cleaning as our brain is on top of its game, leaving us feeling less tired and more focused on what we want out of life.

The Good Outweighs the Bad

After all my teasing, I think it's about time we get down to business and list some of the specific advantages (and risks). Not all of us have the time for rambling, after all, so here we go:

Some Good Adam's Ale

Water is an excellent, all-natural supplement if you're taking up a sport or if you start exercising. This might be great for you, especially if you don't already have the second simple habit tucked under the belt. When we exercise, we sweat and lose a lot of electrolytes (and we dehydrate quicker).

When we drink water, we return everything we lost on the field or gym floor—drinking electrolyte-rich drinks further replenishes what we lose in sodium. There's more. While we're active, getting in some water helps lower the body temperature, increases brainpower and energy, builds muscle, and even puts more *oomph* into your ticker!

In short, you'll amp up your overall performance and health, all while snatching up that extra mile you need to stay motivated to do one more push-up or shoot for another point.

Best of all, water does all of it with or without exercise. Although, exercise is something you have to include in your life if you want to be healthy and happy. Still, from stabilizing your heartbeat to balancing electrolytes or pumping oxygen to your cells, water does it all and more!

While we're on the topic of exercising, another popular new year's resolution many of us have embraced at least once is shedding some pounds. Water is a splendid weight loss aid as it fills you up and replaces all those sugary drink calories we get from sodas, alcohol, coffee, and juices.

Furthermore, water helps with a problem many of us suffer from: a lowered or slow metabolism. When you reach a specific age, I swear it just goes downhill! There's some good news, though. According to the University of Washington, drinking a glass of cold water helps to increase metabolism (Amidor, 2021). Even though it's only by a little bit, it's said to help you burn an added eight calories per day! So, why not slim down simply by throwing some ice in a glass with some fresh water?

Then there's nursing your digestion (and fighting off constipation), protecting all your organs and tissues, and even adding some cushion to your joints! I can go on and on, but clearly there's an endless script of the advantages to drinking more water.

Now imagine how much you'll flourish once drinking water has become a habit! I know it might sound strange and possibly a hard thing to do for some. However, with a little practice, it's not so bad. Once you've learned some tips and tricks and stick to them, you'll learn all of the ins and outs in no time, and before you can say H^2O, you'll have some water ready to go!

Risky Business

I'll be running through what happens when we don't drink enough water rather quickly, because a lot (and enough) negativity is going around these days. However, I'm not skipping this because you must know the risks you run from neglecting the blue. I've come across multiple people in my career who "want" change but still don't fully commit to specific steps they would have to take, such as drinking water in this case. Sometimes, all they need is a so-called jump-scare and some tough love.

Here are some of the risks:

1. throbbing headaches from dehydration (painkillers won't help)
2. hard stools and constipation (which no one wants)
3. dry and ashy skin that has no glow or radiancy, plumpness, or elasticity
4. fatigue and brain fog
5. weight gain (we sometimes mistake hunger cues for thirst)
6. lack of saliva which leaves you with a dry mouth (and sometimes stinky breath)
7. dehydration (which, as previously mentioned, could even kill you.)
8. possibly catching mild to severe illnesses as your immune system is weakened (which is a gamble you shouldn't want to take)

So, either get ready for some consecutive bad days, sick-times, and unhealthy "vibes" (because that's where a lack of water gets you), or it's about time to step up to the plate and grab that glass!

HOW MUCH IS ENOUGH

According to the Mayoclinic, the average human should drink between 91.2979 fl oz and 125.112 fl oz (nearly a gallon), including the water you get from other beverages and food (2020). The first number is the advised amount for women, and the higher amount is for men.

It might seem a lot at first, but it isn't that much of a stretch once you get used to drinking water daily. You should also remember how much water you lose daily through going to the loo (sounds so British!) and essential everyday things such as breathing.

Some people might even require a bit more depending on their lifestyle and surroundings. A person that lives in warmer climates and exercises, for example, will require a bit more than the recommended amount to ensure that their body works just right.

Finding Balance

When gauging how much water you'll have to gulp down, you start by estimating your *Total Daily Energy Expenditure (TDEE)*. I know, what is that even?! Simply put, it's how much energy you use in a single day. Once you know this, you'll be able to sum up how much water you'll need to keep your body going.

The overall amount of water you should drink within a day falls close to the average recommendation. However, several other factors and determinators come into play, such as your age, gender, body mass, activity level, and the climate.

Lucky for us, with the age of technology at the door, we've got quite the resources, various apps, and nearly infinite websites at our hands. Numerous online calculators form part of this support net, which allows you to grasp what the right amount of water you should drink could look like.

Nevertheless, you shouldn't immediately follow the first calculator you stumble upon, as some are more accurate than others. My advice would be to try out a few of them, mark down all of the results you got, and then choose one of two options. Your best shot would be to go with the amount that comes up more than once or go for the highest fl oz you get. Although, if you choose to go for the second option, you'll still have to do some further digging to make sure you're not "overdrinking" and that the amount you've settled on is still safe.

However, my sleeves aren't empty. You can start with this simple calculation so as not to confuse yourself and have some sort of jumping board. I do still recommend that you do some further self-studying and digging since this calculator only includes two factors out of many others. Weight and activity level. So, when you get the time, definitely start calculating some answers of your own and go from there!

1. Take your weight (in lbs).
2. Multiply your weight by 2/3.
3. Work at your activity level.
4. For every 30 minutes you exercise, add 12 oz.

Thus, if we look at an example, it would look more or less like this:

Jane is 55 years old, and she weighs 132.28 lbs. She exercises 45 minutes per day. Also, she lives in southern Florida, which has a higher tropical climate.

Her calculation would start with her weight, which we know is 132.28 lbs. Multiply that by 2/3, and you get 88.9 fl oz. Since we know that she exercises 45 minutes a day, there would be 18 oz added on top of her initial amount (12 oz for 30 minutes and 6 oz for the remaining 15 minutes).

Then we blend everything together, and we're left with 106.9, or rounded up to 107 oz, for the amount of water Jane should be drinking.

Although, when we glimpse at Jane's age and where she lives, we know that she would be taking in more water to compensate for the heat and other problems. As we get older, our body temperature changes (along with other things such as our weakened joints, skin elasticity, etc.). Thus she will have to drink more water to help her as she ages (beautifully, might I add). For women, this is around the age where they could have stepped into menopause, which will definitely require more water. There will be a lot going on, and her body temperature will skyrocket!

She could also be on some medication, which could mean she should be drinking more water or, in some cases, less water, such as with certain heart medications.

Note how I said sometimes medication could mean that she should actually slow down on her water? Well, that's because there are cases where less is more.

I know—I keep hammering on about drinking a lot of water, and now here I am again, telling you that maybe you could be overdrinking. Since we're trying to make a habit of drinking water, I'm presuming that this is not the case. Although it definitely can be. With this, your focus will have to lie in doubling down, keeping a closer eye on your intake, and taking a step back. Overall, with enough water, too little, or too much, the habit is more or less the same: drinking water while staying true to your health.

Drowning yourself in water should already hoist a red flag to you, and that's because it is. As mentioned, drinking water while taking certain medications isn't the best of ideas. One reason is that it could lead to you holding onto all the water you drank.

Water retention doesn't sound like fun because it isn't fun. There are two ways it can go: Water retention could mean there are some hidden health conditions you should look at. However, if it's a case of overdrinking, there are things you could do that could get you back on track, such as reducing your salt intake and moving around more.

When you overdrink water and your body holds most of it in, there are a lot of tell-signs and consequences that follow:

- You have a headache that nothing can soothe.
- Nausea (and yes, of course, vomiting) torments you, and if that's not enough, you'll be getting up constantly to get to the bathroom.

- You'll experience swollen limbs, primarily hands, and feet, as well as your lips.
- (The next one, I personally love to blame, especially after a long holiday) Retained water can cause a bloated stomach and some added water weight.
- You'll feel even more tired, this time with some weak and shaky muscles to match.
- Things can get foggy as you get confused and disoriented because of the sodium in your body taking a steep drop.
- Because the salt within your body is diluted, you could get really sick with hyponatremia.

So, we are again faced with the same question: How much water is enough?

Using the calculators is a great start. Couple that with some safeguards, such as exercising, and you could avoid the whole pesky overdrinking-water-retention thing.

Still, a quick way to make sure that you're on the right path—you'll have to do something that might be strange for some to do—is to take a look at your pee. There's a fine line between yellow and clear that is ideal.

Bright yellow, orange, reddish, or brown urine is a no. This could mean that you're dehydrated, ill, or on medication. This also goes for other colors and hues of urine because there are a lot of variations, surprisingly. Then again, completely clear urine is also a bad thing since this is usually how you can tell you have to cut back on the glasses.

You should aim for pale yellow. That's all, a hint of yellow in the bowl or the urinal, making sure that it's not always clear waters, but also not some strange colored lakes.

JILL'S TROUBLES

(I know this might be uncomfortable for some, but it's normal, and I'm sure almost all of you have experienced the same thing…)

Jill has been backed-up. Constipated. Has been for five days. Which is a long time not to go to the bathroom. Jill also thought so, so she went to her doctor. His prescription was simple, "Drink more water!"

So that's what she did: She increased her consumption by 38.44 fl oz, *et voila*. Within no time, she was galloping to the bathroom. Now, Jill knows that not drinking enough water will cause her to get bunged up, and she has an all-natural remedy she could use whenever the future calls for it!

GET-UP-AND-GO

Sometimes we all could use some motivation. Earlier I told you that motivation doesn't last, and I still firmly believe that that's the case. However, incentives could go a long way when trying to turn something you rarely or never did into your day-to-day routine. Habits aren't something we are born with. Even when we learn habits as babies, we memorize steps and actions before carrying them as habits (you already know this, as I've probably blabbered this over a dozen times by now).

In a nutshell, motivation pushes the boulder up the hill, then once the habit is at the top and set in stone, you can rest assured you've crested the summit.

Ways to Motivate

1. Getting in the right amount of fluids can get tricky. Thus, slamming a big bottle of water next to you could help you remember to gulp some down every now and then.

Advice alert: invest in an insulated or tumbler-style water bottle to keep water cold (especially for bigger bottles), and throw in some ice.

2. For all the water-haters out there, I told you I've got something to help. Add flavor to your water. There are various "make-it-yourself" choices and variations, like adding lemon juice, cucumbers, or strawberries. Then there are also some "water infusions" you can look around for and buy if needed. I once bought some watermelon drops, and it turned out pretty great.

3. If you still find you're forgetting to hydrate, set yourself reminders (such as alarms on your phone, sticky notes on your desk, or ask a friend to send you a text!).

4. Set up challenges for yourself to complete, such as drinking a certain amount of glasses before lunch. You could, for example, even drag a friend or family member into the match to see who drank their required amount of water the most within a week or month—something engaging and fun to spice up your motivation (and accountability).

5. When starting out, you could rotate your drinks. Drink water, then soda, then some water, and you get my point. Although, this shouldn't become your standard routine, as most drinks like this still are bad for your health. The best would be to drown out these beverages with some water as you progress.

6. Another great way to shape drinking water into a habit is to stick it with other habits within your routine. Such as drinking water once you get out of bed, before and after meals, and other times like that.

7. Keeping track of your water intake is a great way to record how much water you're drinking. All while having a blast (well, it's fun for me, at least). There are various

ways you could record your intake and progress, the method and medium being entirely up to you.

8. My personal favorite is keeping a journal. I start with the date on the top before I draw hideous attempts of empty glasses. Usually, my doodled containers represent 17 fl oz. After drinking that amount, I strike a line through the glass or "fill" in the water with some ink. It helps me unwind while I'm working, and when I get home, I know how much water I've had during the day and how much I still have to chug. Journals also don't have to be physical. You can always keep a journal digitally using a notepad or Word processing tool or app.

9. Various applications were specifically made to help you keep track of how much water you drank. Some apps also include features that send you reminders when it's time to refill, kicking out the previous incentive technique of reminding yourself. I'm confident I can't mention them by name, but the best would be to surf the web and your app store, try some out, and find one that works for you.

10. The last motivational tip is short and sweet: *Do you*. There's nothing wrong with experimenting with strategies, changing things up, and finding your own ways to motivate. It's called self-motivation, after all. To share a quick example story, a lady I knew tried to drink water strictly, but she also treasured her wine. Hence, she came up with a sort of "self-trickery" method where she would still have her wineglass in her hand at the end of the night, but instead of filling it with grapes, she stuck with ice cubes and water. What can I say? If it works, it works, even when it might sound and look silly!

That's all I have to say. So, hydrate and stick with these motivational tactics until the water bottle is habitually swallowed up and held high above your crown! As Jim Ryun said, "Motivation is what gets you started. Habit is what keeps you going" (Duff, 2021).

Hydrated Worksheet

Keeping a "worksheet" of some sort to keep track of your progress is really helpful when creating habits. When it comes to drinking water, recording your intake will help you see how much water you drank in a day and how close you are to knocking it in as a goal. You'll see how your progress is growing and how independent you're getting from the constant reminders to drink one more glass.

For example, If you start with a dozen reminders, tracking nonstop, forgetting a few times, etc. Then one day, you go to record 17 oz, and you find that, even though you have no reminder, you've actually drunk 51 oz already. You just forget to jot down the other two glasses. Still, you did drink that water, and you did so without thinking and overthinking about it! That's where we want to go. The key is to stay on top of your game until drinking water becomes a habit and you see the results you've been plunging towards.

Journaling or simply answering worksheets are great ways to wrap your mind around what you're doing, how it's going, and what needs to be done. Here's a quick run-through example of what your worksheet could end up like. Why not give it a try?!

The H²O Tracker	
GOAL (Oz):	**Date(s):**
Track your water here (whichever way you like):	

The H²O Q's
Why do you want to make drinking water a habit in your life?
Did you make your intake-amount goal? If not, why do you think that is? Did you drink more than your goals? Why do you think that is?
Was it hard or easy or hard for you to drink the amount of water?
What motivational strategy did you use? Did it work for you? Are you sticking with one, or are you going to try another? If yes, which one is your next go-to?

The H²O Q's
Was there anything you think you could've done better or different today?
What will you change tomorrow?
How did you feel after drinking this much water today? Did you notice any changes in your body (less tired, lower temperature,etc.) How was your mood?

The H²O Q's
(Important) Did you notice any triggers? List them. How did you handle them? How will you fight them? How will you turn these triggers around to benefit you and your goals?

5

COUNTING SHEEP

Let her sleep, for when she wakes, she will shake the world.
–Napoleon Bonaparte

We all know what sleep is because we do it every day—or night, usually. Whether or not we have good sleeping patterns is another story. We've all been told that a good eight hours is enough time to catch up on some z's and feel happy go lucky, and all that stuff.

Well, forget what you've been told, as the amount of sleep a person needs could depend on various things. Most adults fall under the seven to nine hours mark, while older folks only need seven to eight. Children need more sleep (thankfully) than the adults taking care of them, up to 12 hours if they're under 12 and up to 16 hours as infants. In some cases, however, you might need more or less sleep, such as when a woman is pregnant and she requires several more hours of sleep to protect, nurture, and grow her baby.

When we doze off, our bodies go through four stages of sleep.

These four stages can go on for several minutes, multiple times in a single sitting:

- Stage 1: A light sleep where everything slows down.
- Stage 2: Still sleeping lightly, but bodily function begins to slow or drop (like your breathing rate or body temperature). Your body relaxes more until you fall into a deep sleep.
- Stage 3: This is where your deep sleep starts; where you "sleep like a rock." Your eyes and muscles don't move, and your brain waves slow down. This phase makes you feel more awake and refreshed once you wake up.
- Stage 4: This phase is where your *Rapid Eye Movement (REM)* sleeping takes over. Your brain activity increases, your eyes dart around (hence the name), and you start dreaming. This is also the phase where the brain processes information, taking everything you've learned during the day and filing it into your long-term memory.

No one really understands what role certain sleep stages play biologically, besides resetting the physical system (such as allowing ample time for muscular repair). Still, various research and studies have shown that sleep majorly impacts our cardiovascular system, immune system, and metabolism. Your entire body shifts into change-overdrive when you sleep, and with this, changes are definitely good. Sleep, in essence, is the perfect protein shake to keep your body in tip-top shape so it can function at its very best!

WHAT A DREAM

Well, let's not sit around wasting daylight, shall we? Why don't we jump right into some ways that sleep just... works!

Busy Brains

One would think that when you're fast asleep, your brain also takes some time off to relax and unwind. However, it's quite the opposite. When the curtains fall, this is when our brains get even busier!

We now know that while we get some shut-eye, we run through four stages of sleep. With these levels, researchers thought that it would be a good idea to measure brain waves; they did so and noted down the clear patterns our brains took while going through these changes. There were slow and steady swirls to quick bursts of energetic stirs. This observation made things a bit clearer (for the researchers, anyway!). Our brains metaphorically run around, climb the walls, and slide all over our skulls, doing what it has to do while the body is the one that gets the time out.

As noted a few lines up, sleep helps us manage everything. It moves what we've learned and experienced during the day to our "long-term file cabinets," locking them in for good. Our brains even do a bit of housekeeping while they're at it! This means that we could learn more later.

There are 24 hours in a day, and a lot could happen within that time, good or bad. Regardless of toxicity, these thoughts, experiences, feelings, responses, and stressors—they pile up. Thus, once your head hits the pillow, it's your brain's job to remove the clutter such as needless info and recollections, to make sure you wake up with a clear head that works well.

I have a theory. Well, I don't have one *per se*. It was psychologist William James who did, and he called it the theory of *brain plasticity*.

I know, about now you're probably thinking, *No! no more, Kate, please! We're getting pretty technical here!!* Just sit tight; the theory isn't as formidable or complex as it sounds. It's a way to explain the way your brain's glymphatic system takes all the rubble from your head, ties it up in a garbage bag, and then tosses it out from your central nervous system. It's almost like your brain is spring cleaning while you're asleep, which is great.

Once you're awake, some aspects of your brain are affected, even when you don't notice them. Such as your:

- information processing and learning
- memory (short-term and long-term)
- problem-solving skills
- creativity
- focus and concentration
- ability to make decisions

Overall, your brain is just more alive, awake, and active when you wake up. That is, if you slept well and for long enough. Thus, everything your brain has worked on through the night will work better: You can collect more data and store more memories while your increased brainpower and energy will have you doing more throughout your day. A clearer mind also allows you to walk around with some footing on your emotions, thoughts, and feelings. However, I'll temporarily hush about that since the next heading is short on our heels!

The Feels

Has anyone ever told you that you're not thinking "clearly" or being "unreasonable"? If you get enough sleep, you can point out that they're wrong! Well, in most cases, anyway. This is because you're thinking on your toes and dealing with emotions more logically. So, hopefully, there will be fewer mood swings and exasperation with the people around you (although no amount of sleep can kill how annoying you might find some people).

Emotions are reigned in on a good night's sleep, allowing you to grip, control, and manage them more securely. How, you ask?

There are areas in our brains that keep our emotions in check. Because they're flooded with surges of activity, they work better. This is a great booster shot for your emotional health and stability, as well as proper, healthy brain functioning. When you get enough sleep, you'll be able to adapt and respond to certain situations in a better way.

There are quite a few areas of the brain where these activities increase, and yes, most of them sound quirky, fancy, hard to pronounce, and... Well, you'll see what I mean:

- *Amygdala: This part of the brain is responsible for screaming "Danger! Danger!" whenever we stumble upon something that we either find suspicious or scary; it helps us regulate our emotions and is responsible for activating our fight or flight responses.*
- *Striatum:* Motor and action planning, motivation, decision-making, reinforcement, and reward perception live here.
- *Hippocampus:* Learning, emotional response, memory formation, and storage of memories can be found in this region.
- *Insula:* This is where taste, visceral sensation, and autonomic control originate; the insula also regulates the immune system
- *Medial Prefrontal Cortex (mPFC)*: Mingles with different parts of our brain to stockpile and process memories, which links to the formation of habits. The mPFC is also known to oversee our inhibitions, impulses, and how we pay attention.

On that note, I should mention that there's usually not just one part that does only one thing within our brains; most components play and work together, doing the same things and puppeteering us around to do whatever we do.

Sometimes, certain situations pop up that we aren't sure how to handle. This is where our amygdalas could be high-jacked, causing our emotions to burst! These situations don't come along that often, but they are more likely to happen when we're tired. Being well-rested means that response is handled in a more adaptive and reasonable *manière* (way). You'll seem calm and collected (which you will be), while all it took was some bedtime. In the same way, the other parts of your brain are pushed forward, ensuring that you're always one step ahead of any situation life throws your way.

Hormones and Strong Bones

While we're asleep, our bodies open the floodgates for hormones to release into our bodies. Don't worry, though. All is still good in the body department, as all the hormones mean well and serve a purpose.

There are hormones released while you sleep to help you sleep —well, obviously, *something* in your body has to have that magic. In this case, it's a tiny pea-shaped gland in the brain called the pineal gland. This gland is what controls your sleeping patterns and produces a hormone called melatonin to help make sleeping more comfortable. In all honesty, it sounds like a bread spread to me! Or maybe I'm just hungry.

Apart from pumping into your body natural sleeping meds, the pineal gland releases growth hormones. Which does what it says, helps you grow (and repair).

You see, sleeping is like an auto repair shop: Your body is the screeching car that teeters over to spend the night in the old greasy garage. In the same way that our cars have to go in for maintenance and repairs, our bodies have to undergo some work from time to time, and they do so by sleeping. Muscles, tissues, and cells are restored when our bodies release all sorts of hormones and proteins. Everything gets fixed and waxed up in a wink! And all it took was a quick nap.

This wholesome process will undoubtedly come in handy once you start hitting the gym (or home gym) since sore muscles are the worst. Sleeping, coupled with this process, steps in to heal and soothe us right up!

Your metabolism will also get a kick from this, which will help you ditch some weight and keep it off. All while controlling your appetite, thanks to some more hormones called leptin and ghrelin. Which, at first, just sounded like the stars of some sort of 90s mystical creature horror flick.

While sleeping, you'll also notice that your hormone production during the day is more effective.

Medicinal Mattresses

I haven't slammed down the locks on hormones just yet, because there's still one hormone I would like to bring up, and I think it's one you may already know about: insulin.

If you've heard the name and don't know what it is, or you've never even heard of it before, think about diabetes. Once again, the same goes for that definition. Diabetes is an illness where a person's insulin levels aren't as they should be, either having too little in the body or too much. This will result in the body not knowing how to process glucose, or sugar, within the body, making the person very ill.

Although sleep can't make diabetes vanish, it sure wouldn't hurt. When a diabetic person doesn't sleep enough, insulin levels rise, making it harder for the person to manage their condition. However, many diabetics (including my grandpa) say they struggle to get any sleep. Which is overall just a horrible cycle. Thus, if you are a diabetic and sleeping doesn't come easy to you, I advise you to visit your doctor. The same goes for any of you that suffer from sleep disorders, such as insomnia. If you want to make a habit of sleeping, having these challenges to carry around will make the road even tougher for you to ride out, and might not even work without some medical guidance.

However, if you don't have diabetes, you should still watch out. There are two types of diabetes. Type one is an autoimmune disease and is sometimes inherited, while type 2 diabetes is commonly caused by an unhealthy lifestyle. Where I'm going with this is that you could protect yourself from getting the latter by adding some minutes (or hours) to your sleeping routine. This is because sleep keeps your cells healthy, and cells are the little guys who take up glucose and use it to regulate the overall glucose count in the blood.

While we're on the medicinal mattress of it all, I want to move on to something we all know, that one thing that steps between us and all sorts of ailments. That's right, our immune system. (I felt like Dora the Explorer there.) Sleep has been proven to affect our immunity's ability to fight off germs, illnesses, and infections.

Infections and inflammation are no child's play, and our bodies know that. This is why they leak out proteins called cytokines. While making these fun-sounding proteins, the body also puts together new antibodies and immune cells. You're left almost brand-new!

Sleep coupled with all these hormonal, protein-laced ingredients makes for the perfect flu pack—destroying any harmful germs in its way!

Take a look at when we're tired, and obviously, the complete opposite happens. Our bodies weaken, leaving us more vulnerable to germs and illnesses.

Remember how your mom always told you to get sleep when

you felt a bit under the weather? It was because your body needed it to be healthy again. Sleeping away will also help you target your stress, symptoms of depression, and prevent seizures, high blood pressure, and all those more-than-fine-without migraines.

On top of that, not getting enough sleep has also been linked to heart diseases and risk factors, such as high blood pressure, elevated cortisol, etc. All of this means your ticker is getting the short end of the stick, not to mention how fatal it could be to your health. In contrast to what's been said, sleeping enough could make your heart fitter and your stress (cortisol) levels a lot dimmer.

Clearly, sleeping by itself is medicine—a personal first aid kit built into your circadian rhythm! It contributes enormously to your health in various ways (and yes, you best believe I only mentioned a slight lick of benefits!). Sleep really balances you out while you're in dreamland, and as established before—it's all about balance!

PROBLEMS WITH A 'Z'

Weighing in at 100 pounds of everything rotten! Standing in the Everybody-has-those-nights corner! The one, the only, *I can't sleep!*

You were probably able to tell by that horrendous introduction that I'm in the same boat as you probably are: It's currently 11 p.m., and I'm still wide awake. The thing is, I've got sleeping as a habit under control, so why?!

Well, because everyone has those nights where no amount of tossing and turning, habit or not, can put you to sleep. I think it's noteworthy for you to know this as you're taking on the habit. It won't always be, "On your marks, get set, and go! to sleep..." Things happen, and all you have to do is not let them get to you.

One night of going to bed late or just being restless is all it takes to make you feel horrible, though. I know I'll be feeling it tomorrow! Still, there's a simple cure: sleep. You'll be back to your old, energetic self in no time. This might throw off your habit a bit, so try and stick with the sleeping routine as best you can while creating the new pattern.

What might happen if you went a night without sleep? Sleeping is, as we've come to know, very essential in our day-to-day lives—and by day-to-day, I mean *every single day*. As pulmonologist and sleep disorder specialist Samuel Gurevich explains, "Sleeping is important because being awake is important, and one or two nights of bad sleep can impair your ability to function well for the next day" (Cleveland Clinic, 2021).

He meant that even just a single night of going to bed a bit later than usual can have serious consequences. I can tell you this much; by tomorrow, I'll definitely experience at least one of these effects:

- irritability
- sleepiness
- slower reaction time
- lack of concentration and focus
- problems with remembering things
- anxiety or depression

Some of these might not seem all that bad. I mean. One cup of coffee (even though I'm trying to cut back) is enough to make me more awake and less irritable. So? Problem solved! Not quite. If you take a closer look, you'll see that you're putting yourself right in harm's way. Your attention, focus, concentration, and reaction time are limited. Which is a recipe for disaster! Imagine driving to work with your eyes glued shut and your ears stuffed with corks. Not fun, right? Well, that's what you're in for if you lack all of these things (just go with the image.) You might even think, "I've got this," but the chances are, you don't.

Now you probably think I'm a hypocrite since I've just told you a whole story about how I was staying up late and that old tale.

Well, no one's perfect. Besides, I'm already tucked into bed, ready to turn another sheet. Still, don't worry too much if you find that you can't sleep well—so long as it's only a night or two.

This often happens when we're stressed or faced with some things that keep our minds busy. Our bodies usually recover quickly from these few bursts of restlessness. It's going over a day or two you should be worried about because that's really when our bodies start feeling the blows!

I don't want to get all negative on you because, let's face it, the good is so much sweeter! Then again, it doesn't matter what I think since there can't be good without the bad. That might be misleading—let me rephrase: If you have a good sleeping routine, you can get all the good you can carry. Still, just hear me out.

What a Nightmare

We know that without enough sleep, our bodies get messy. Nevertheless, let's run through all the things that go bump in the night (when you don't sleep):

- increased risk of early death
- stronger feelings of pain
- lowered sex drive
- wrinkled skin, dark circles under the eye
- hallucinations

WHERE YOU STAND

The Sleep Foundation defines sleep deprivation as a general term for when you "don't get the sleep you need," (Suni, 2022).

I've come across many people who believe that sleep deprivation is only used to describe sleepless nights related to underlying diseases, such as sleep apnea. However, this isn't the case. If you take the word "deprived" on its own, it's defined as a "lacking something that is needed," such as sleep (Cambridge Dictionary, 2019). Thus, you don't have to have an illness to be sleep-deprived; elements such as stress, strain because of educational or career requirements, and poor sleeping habits could all contribute to those restless nights.

Common signs that you might be sleep-deprived:

- feeling drowsy and falling asleep during the day
- falling asleep within five minutes of lying down
- microsleeps during waking hours
- having a hard time getting out of bed
- mood changes
- forgetfulness
- sleeping more on days when you don't have the alarm clock set

The quickest way to self-evaluate whether or not you're getting in enough sleep is to ask yourself:

- Do you feel that your sleep schedule is proper, adequate, and healthy?
- Do you sleep enough to be productive and get everything done throughout the day?
- Do you feel sleepy or find yourself dozing off during the day?
- Do you rely on caffeine (coffee, tea, energy drinks,) to give you energy during the day?
- Would you say you have a fairly regular sleeping pattern? Meaning you wake up and go to sleep even on weekends, holidays, and any other "off" days.

Whether your results came back as "you might be sleep-deprived," or "you most definitely are," there's no need to freak out. There are some ways you could get some "self-treatment" unless you feel you need medical care, in which case you need to stop by the doctor. Also, it's advised that if you snore chronically and loudly, stop breathing periodically while asleep, experience daytime irritability or sleepiness (especially after sleeping), and/or have trouble falling asleep no matter what you do, you should also see a medical professional (Haines, 2022).

As for self-treatment, there are a few things you can try to make going to bed more effortless, the most crucial way is taking a look at your sleeping schedule and deciding whether or not something could change. You can also avoid certain things before bed, and take on some tips and tricks in your life—don't worry, I've got them in spades. So, why don't we get down to business?

THE SLEEPING PILL

Various things in a day clash with how we sleep at night, such as what we eat and drink, the medication we take, certain activities, and the times we do them. Everything influences everything. It's important to understand that so you can change your sleeping patterns while establishing some groundbreaking habits. Which, as a fun fact, is called having good "sleep hygiene."

So, the best way to ensure your sleep hygiene is under control is to create a regular and stable sleeping schedule. This commonly means setting an early bedtime that gives you at least seven to eight or nine hours of sleep (as explained before) and a specific time to wake up. Then all that's left to do is stick with those times, no matter if it's the weekend, holiday, and days like those.

This, of course, is easier said than done. There are, however, small things we can do to ensure that our new and improved way of sleeping becomes easier to do.

First of all, take some safety measures and actions awhile before you go to bed:

- Limit your exposure to bright light in the evening.
- Make sure to hit the off button at least 30 minutes before bed.
- Avoid drinking caffeine in the afternoon and evening (that's why most people refer to it as "morning coffee").
- If you plan on exercising in the afternoon, make sure to do so two to three hours before bed.
- Reduce your fluids so that you won't get up every five minutes to go to the bathroom, and any alcohol before bed is a definite no.
- Also, try not to eat any heavy meals. If you're really past-starving hungry, go for a light and healthy snack if you have to.
- Make sure that your bedroom is as comfortable as it can be, keeping the room temperature cool and relaxed, and also just using the bedroom for all those bedroom activities (such as sleeping and *you-know-what*) so that your brain can make and keep a connection between the two.

Furthermore, opt for a relaxing bedtime routine. This can, for example, be something like exercising a few hours before bedtime, then taking a relaxing bath, then doing some crossword puzzles at the dining room table, or reading a book in the armchair until you're feeling sleepy—thereafter you actually go to bed, try not to fall asleep on the couch or at your desk. Doing some sort of boring activity before bed is a great way to tire you out, and not going to bed unless you're feeling sleepy is great to avoid creating some sort of dramatic, obsessive scenario in your head and things like that.

Also, if you're in bed and you notice that after 20 minutes, you're getting nowhere in terms of sleeping, get up and go do some boring stuff!

These are just simple (yet effective) ways you can make the chances of falling asleep fall in your favor. However, there are countless other ways to help you make your sleeping pattern better or help you fall asleep on those bad, restless nights. This can be anything from getting into yoga, meditation, or mindfulness, avoiding naps during the day, keeping an eye on what you consume, practicing writing to soothe your anxiety and stress, trying aromatherapy, or something as simple as focusing on trying to stay awake while in bed, or thinking happy thoughts.

Now, of course, you don't have to throw in all of these things—although, it wouldn't hurt to do some of them, such as cutting out the electronics and light—but try to focus on unwinding, eating lighter meals before bed, and balanced meals in general (although that's a habit for another day).

Restless Ruth

Ruth was never someone who skipped sleep, and when she did sleep, she slept like a baby. Then, out of nowhere, she started waking up in the middle of the night and no matter how hard she tried she couldn't press snooze on her insomnia. Hours would pass, and just when she would doze off, her alarm would scream.

Night after night, this went on and she started feeling exhausted and emotionally burned out, her appetite went down the drain, and brain fog became a part of her day. She started to feel terrible and self-conscious, while all the people that constantly kept noting how she looked older and telling her that she could do it with a quick 20 winks, sure didn't help.

She had no idea what was going on. That was until she noticed that it was her lack of sleep that was to blame. Even worse, she knew it was becoming a habit. She knew she had to take action!

She opted to break her habit by giving herself a few nights to sleep it off! Just a night or two to get accustomed to how good it felt to sleep in, and kind of trick herself into wanting more.

In her case, she started off by taking a natural sleeping aid (I don't want to encourage any drug-taking, which is why I haven't mentioned it before, but please, if this is what you think would work, go all-natural like drinking chamomile tea, or seek proper medical advice and supervision; and don't become dependent on this, make sure to gradually replace the aid with more natural habits).

After just two nights of sleeping like a log, Ruth knew that she had to have this all the time! So, consciously she made the decision to press for a good night's rest every night by making it a habit. And you know what... She did it!

Sure, periodically she'll have a rough night where she can't sleep. But as was said earlier, it happens to everyone. Besides, it never lasts longer than a night or two because she caps the bad habit and quickly replaces it with a good one instead. She even ditched the natural aid after a few nights and replaced it with the *4-7-8 breathing method.*

You know I'm here for you so if you're interested, the 4-7-8 breathing technique as developed by Dr. Andrew Weil, is below:

1. Place the tip of your tongue behind your upper front teeth.
2. Exhale through your mouth. It should make a sort of whoosh, frustrated snake-type sound (you'll see what I mean when you do it).
3. Close your mouth. Inhale through your nose while counting (not out loud) to four.
4. Hold that breath and count to seven.
5. Place the tongue back behind your teeth and exhale (along with the whoosh) and count to eight.

6. Repeat this whole process at least three more times.

Snoozin'

Keeping track of how many hours you're sleeping is a great way to not only keep you motivated to stick to your schedule but also to see how much sleep you're getting, how much you still need, and so on—so if you can track it, why not?

The most common way to track your sleep these days would be to get some sort of wearable device, such as a smartwatch or sleeping pad. They are more accurate than you guessing or estimating the time you sleep, when you go to sleep, and when you wake up, because, as we know by now, sleep isn't that simple.

The thing is, that is a way you can more or less try and figure out how long you're sleeping since some of these devices can get a bit pricey. But, if you're willing to invest, the best you can do is go through all the available devices out there, scan through a bunch of reviews and complaints, and then decide which one would work for you best (with your budget in mind, of course).

YAWNING REFLECTIONS

Think about your sleep routine and complete the reflection diary (SLE Education, n.d.):

What activities do you do before sleeping?

What is something that distracts you from sleeping?

What's something that helps you sleep better?

When was the last time you had a good night's rest?

At what time do you go to sleep?

At what time do you wake up?

You could sleep better if you...

How do you feel after sleeping well vs. after a night of not sleeping too well?

Do this activity as often as you like, whether it's a daily sign-in, a weekly review, or a monthly check-in, just make sure to answer these questions from time to time, while also adding in some other questions, such as "How has my sleeping routine and schedule changed?" and, "How do I feel today compared to x (days/weeks/months) ago?"

6

YOU ARE WHAT YOU EAT

To eat is a necessity, but to eat intelligently is an art.
–François de la Rochefoucauld

We need a healthy plate of food to have a balanced diet that can give our bodies all the nutrients they need to work efficiently. Without healthy eating habits, we are more prone to illnesses, diseases, and other conditions; we gain weight, feel like hell, and— well, nothing good comes from eating badly. Overall, balanced eating is the way to go. As they (and the heading) say, *you are what you eat*.

As we've established, water is absorbed. Food, on the other hand, is digested. From there, food is sent to all the other parts of our bodies, such as the pancreas and liver, where juices are made to ship the food to your smaller intestines.

This is, once again, where most of the nutrients are pulled from your food and passed along for the body to use or store. Cells help absorb the nutrients into your bloodstream, where simple sugars, amino acids, glycerol, vitamins, and salts are sent to the liver. This is where the nutrients are stored, processed, and delivered to the rest of your body where needed.

Your body has a network of vessels, the *lymphatic system*, which carries white blood cells and a fluid called lymph throughout the body to fight infections and absorb fatty acids and vitamins. All of these nutrients, in the end, are also used to build substances you need for growth, energy, and cellular repairs.

With all that quickly cleared out of the way, the question still remains: Why do we need proper nourishment?

LET'S TACO 'BOUT IT?

Did your mom ever go on about how you "had to" eat your vegetables, or else this and that would happen? Well, mine sure did. And even though I can't quite remember what those "dire consequences" were, I know that her heart meant well because here I am today, mothering you about how you should be eating. Although, I promise that all of this moaning and lecturing will be worth it.

As I've mentioned, when we don't have healthy eating patterns, we're more likely to get sick. As an idea of the severity, the Center for Science in the Public Interest stated that four of the top ten leading causes of death in the US are directly linked to our diets. These are heart diseases, cancers, strokes, and type 2 diabetes (Migala, 2020). Poor nutrition is the leading cause of these diseases. Your immune system will also be weaker, leading to other severe and less severe illnesses and you'll get sicker more often than someone who eats wholesome plates of food. Basically, all of these habits are a part of that "first aid kit" I mentioned before.

Good nutrition will also help keep you healthy mentally, as vitamins and minerals have been shown to prevent mental disorders, such as depression, from rising in our heads. Thus, you're getting a full-body clean-up, polish, and boost. And who doesn't want that!

As a part of the full-body package, there are also a few other add-ins to enjoy:

Recent studies have shown a direct link between eating healthy and upping a person's life expectancy. One study even went as far as to say that by eating healthy, middle-aged adults can add up to seven years to their lifespans (Brown, 2022).

Then there are also the three S's: your skin, smile, and sight. Let's take a look at what nutrients do for you, how to integrate these nutrients into your diet:

Nutrition	What's Its Good For	The Foods (Well, some of them anyway)
Vitamin A	Clears corneas (covering on the outside of the eye) and protects against eye problems (such as cataracts, and age-related macular degeneration or AMD, which causes vision loss).	sweet potatoes, leafy green veggies, bell peppers, and pumpkins
Vitamin B	**B6, B9, B12:** Lower levels of homocysteine, which causes inflammation and increased risk of AMD **B2:** An antioxidant that reduces oxidative stress in the eye and prevents cataracts. **B3:** Can act as an antioxidant and prevents optic nerve damage (or glaucoma). **B1:** Reduces the risk of cataracts, makes for proper cell functioning, and is a potential treatment for early stages of diabetic retinopathy (DR); also, a complication of diabetes that affects the eye and could cause blindness if left untreated.	Further research is required for **B6, B9,** AND **B12** vitamins; studies showed the connection. **B2:** oats, milk, yogurt, beef, and fortified beef **B3:** beef, poultry, fish, mushrooms, peanuts, and legumes
Vitamin C	An antioxidant that protects the eyes against harmful radicals, may benefit those with AMD, and creates collagen (which provides structure to the eyes). Also lowers the risk of developing cataracts.	citrus and other tropical fruits, broccoli, kale, and bell peppers
Vitamin E	An antioxidant that protects eye cells and prevents cataracts	nuts, seeds, cooking oils, salmon, avocadoes, leafy green veggies
Lutein and Zeaxanthin:	Found in the macula and retina of the eye, which helps filter blue light exposure to protect the eyes. Also protects people with cataracts.	cooked spinach, kale, and collard greens
Omega-3 fatty acids	Have anti-inflammatory properties, might prevent DR, and could help those with dry eye diseases.	fish, flaxseed, chia seeds, soy, nuts, walnut- and almond oil

I know, that's a lot to take in, but if you focus on the far right column alone, you'll notice that these are foods you can go out and find at almost any store, it's an easy pickup, so why not go check them out, you'll definitely be able to spot them after all.

Now, as for your chompers. You eat with your teeth, so it would come as logic that your nutrition impacts them directly. Therefore, if you have bad nutrition, you can kiss that smile away, as decay, cavities, and gum disease are on their way!

As every dentist (and probably every toothpaste commercial) would tell you, the best thing you can do to keep your pearls healthy would be to avoid sugars. Although we do have our sweet-tooth people out there, there are some substitutions you can make:

Add fruits to cereal, oatmeal, and low-sugar yogurt. You could also try some honey for all those and your coffee. If it's a hot day outside, try some homemade popsicles, using some fruit, such as pineapple juice and kiwi popsicles. Just like that, you can simply make healthier choices by switching some things around!

A healthy diet can heighten collagen production, which is crucial for skin elasticity and healthy skin cells, while it can also prevent wrinkles from forming, which adds some unneeded years. Having healthy nourishment in your life also means you get some muscle support, strong bones, and a killer digestive system!

The yield of a healthy lifestyle with balanced nutrition is monumental. You will have more energy since you're eating food that gives you more influential nutrients and things for your body to use. Your mood will rise daily, and you will just feel better in general, about your life and yourself.

HERE ARE THE HARSHMALLOWS

The sound of salads, fruit bowls, and "healthy alternatives" is enough to send the majority of the population running for the fried chicken hills! However, hear me out.

The funny thing about life is it sneaks up on you. It never gives you a detailed report or prediction of "what's on for next week!"

Therefore, you can't feel the effects of your bad eating habits... until it's too late. You have to make the changes now and start eating healthy, as it's the only way you can prevent your health from crumbling later. If not for you, then do it for the ones you love. I know, what a clichè! However, in this case, simplicity means truth.

Nobody wants to lose you, especially not when it's too soon. So, eat healthily and stick around for another day! All you have to remember is that "food is not the enemy" (Alicia Galvin, Migala, 2018).

EAT UP! WAIT... HOW MUCH OF WHAT?

There are so many foods out there that are healthy, and I promise you there are just as many of them you either already like or will like once you try them.

There is a very popular image that's replaced the food pyramid of my school days. Think of a plate, and as I'm giving you the recommended amount the food should take these fractions and cut the plate into pieces.

- Vegetables and fruit should take up ½.
- Go colorful and varied (also, remember that potatoes aren't veggies on this plate).
- Whole grains should take up ¼.
- These are whole wheat, barley, wheat berries, quinoa, oats, brown rice, and foods made with them, such as whole wheat pasta (stick with whole and avoid refined).
- Protein should also take up ¼.
- Found in fish, poultry, beans, and nuts are all healthy, versatile protein sources; limit processed and red meats, such as bacon (I know sorry!).
- Go easy on the oils, and rather go for a moderate amount of healthy plant oils, such as olive oil. Avoid hydrogenated oils.

The rest you already have a good idea about. Avoid alcohol, sugary, fatty, and fried foods. While the best shot you have is to do some looking around for healthy foods around you that fit in with your budget and taste. Remember, we live in a world where everything is just a click away, so there are so many varieties and recipes out there for you to try and retry until you find that perfect, nutritious meal plan!

WORDS OF ENCOURAGE-MINTS

The key to getting into some healthy eating habits is to have a fool-proof plan to back you up. There's a lot of temptation out there, fast-food joints around every corner, shelves stacked with snacks and chips, and who knows what else! Thus, you need to have some cold-hard motivation and will to get you through until the habit of eating healthy is all you do!

- Identify your unhealthy eating habits and try replacing them with healthier habits. For example, if you had a habit of carrying candy in your bag or pocket, go for very light, wholesome snacks instead.
- Prepare all your meals beforehand. Make sure your meals are healthy and cut down into smaller portions so that you aren't too full. This will help you stay on track while saving up the money you would have spent on lunch money. Also, it's best to stay away from artificial foods.
- Set reminders for specific times you want to eat so you can stay on some sort of eating schedule and eat slowly, trying to make these sessions last for at least 20 minutes (if possible).
- To keep up on your progress, monitor all of your food choices (in a journal or computer, and you know the rhyme). By monitoring the food choices you make, you

- can know whether you should add some limits, make some changes, or whether you're on the right track.
- Remember what was said way back in the chapters about taking things slow? Well, here baby steps are still in play. However, when it's time for you to go all out, talk with your family, friends, and roommates who live with you about changing up your overall lifestyle by restocking your cabinets. You know what they say, out of sight out of mind, right?
- Most importantly, remember to listen to what your body tells you and what it wants and needs. No matter who says this on whatever website, or who told you they heard what, we all have different bodies that need different things, and you out of all people, know your body the best. So, if you feel like something is tugging where it shouldn't tug, or that something is just feeling off, go see a doctor or dietitian. They can confirm your suspicions and find a better and safer way and diet that will give you the best of what you need.

Oh, Alexandra, Fads Aren't Always Fab

Perhaps to reiterate how we are all different and not one size fits all, we could use Alexandra—who thought that the raw food diet was the way to go to be really healthy. After following it religiously for months on end, she started to gain weight and was feeling anything but healthy, she had bloating issues and lots of stomach aches.

So, she did some allergy testing and found that she had intolerances to cashews, pears, and certain grains, which was what the diet mostly consisted of.

Once she knew this she changed her diet and stopped insisting that all food had to be raw to get the densest nutrient count. She also stopped obsessing about what she was eating all the time and stopped consuming her food with a 'diet' approach completely.

Here she learned the art of listening to her body and not to all the manias out there. She read a beginner's guide to wholesome nutrition and apart from the food she knew she was intolerant to, she ate when she was hungry and what she genuinely felt like eating. She not only felt better, had way more energy, and looked great, but she also started losing extra pounds until eventually she plateaued. She's remained at that healthy weight ever since. Food has become an enjoyment, she often cooks and shares her food with others (known to release more of those feel-good hormones).

A REAL PIZZA-WORK

Where are you eating? *(This can help you see what an impact your environment and scenarios can have on you and your eating habits.)*

What are you doing? And how are you feeling? *(This will help you review your patterns.)*

How hungry are you? *(Before eating the meal, being overly hungry can cause you to overeat.)* You can rate it on a scale, describe it in detail, it's your choice.

What did you "miss" from this meal? *(This can either be something you miss eating, or something that you feel is lacking, such as a bit more fiber.)*

Did you think you ate slowly enough? Did you focus on eating the meal itself or was your thought drifting off somewhere else?

How did you feel after eating? 30 minutes after eating?

Did something go wrong? *(Did you overeat, eat something that wasn't healthy, did you eat more than you could chew, anything like that.)*

7

GYM AND TONIC

If the sun comes up, I have a chance.
–Venus William

Exercise is the missing piece of the puzzle when it comes to drinking water and eating well. It does everything that drinking water and eating healthy do, such as helping you lose weight, and being good for the heart, bones, and muscles while staying fit can also make you live a longer and healthier life.

Furthermore, exercise combats health conditions and diseases, such as strokes, depression (since exercise is also a real mood-booster), metabolic syndromes, etc.

It also helps to foster another habit we've already combed through—sleep. As long as you keep the gap of two to three hours (as mentioned), exercise can be a real sleeping pill on its own. Just like ambient noise, exercising helps soothe our bodies, and since we're balanced, sleep will come more naturally and easier.

I know not everyone is a big fan of running around and pumping iron. However, when you make exercise a regular habit in your life, exercising comes more frequently and smoothly, rather than those small once-in-awhile bursts of activity that don't do a lot. Even just small amounts of exercise every day can make a huge difference!

Aside from that, exercise isn't the painfully dreadful activity it has come to be known of. Exercise can most definitely be something to enjoy. It can help you unwind, get some fresh air, socialize, and just feel good afterward. The key is finding something you enjoy and find comfortable. Zumba classes could make you feel like you're on the next episode of *Dancing With the Stars*, or perhaps you prefer being Louis Armstrong on the bike. The activities you enjoy are more likely to become habits since they aren't forced and you actually look forward to doing them.

DECISIONS, DECISIONS

There are various exercises you can try and take on as a habit. However, most activities can be shaken, stirred, and thrown into four kinds of exercises.

Aerobic Exercises

These are exercises that get your heart pumping and bring your breathing up. These exercises are vital to improving your health and fitness, especially your heart, lungs, and circulatory system, while also giving you that extra mile to do your everyday things. These exercises are also known to slow down and prevent the diseases and health conditions that many older adults experience, such as diabetes, heart diseases, and certain cancers. Here are some examples of aerobic exercises; feel free to give them a try:

- walking (briskly), jogging, and running
- dancing
- swimming

- biking
- hiking/climbing up hills (and even stairs)
- certain sports, such as tennis, basketball, and hockey
- specific exercises, such as jumping rope, mountain climbers, and jumping jacks
- working around the home, such as intensive cleaning and working in the yard, like mowing the lawn and raking the leaves

The US Department of Health and Human Services suggests that, for you to be an average healthy adult, you will need to get in at least 150 minutes (or two and a half hours) worth of moderate aerobic exercise, or 75 minutes (an hour and 15 minutes) of vigorous aerobic exercise, spread along the course of a week. (Wow, that was a mouthful!) While they strongly urge you to do at least 300 minutes (5 hours) worth within a week for the best results in terms of your health.

These are the recommendations, yes. However, not everyone can jump on the track and run their hearts out from the get-go. Thus, know your body and limitations so that you can figure out where you can start off. You can start off doing 30 minutes daily, which will add up to three hours and a half for a week. From there, you can gradually move up to five hours a week, increasing your time and intensity as time goes along and your body improves and gets used to the amount of time and effort you put into this.

Also, why not try and push in as much exercise as you can during your day by doing smaller, quick activities, such as jumping jacks when you wake up, jumping in one spot while you brush your teeth, and using the stairs as much as you can while you're at work?

Strength Training

I know not all of us want to look like some reincarnation of Johnny Bravo, which is more than okay. You don't have to look "buff" to have some healthy muscles tucked away. Still, working on your muscles will be of great benefit to you.

There will be no more days of struggling with the groceries, difficulty getting around, or just trying to do everyday things that require even just a bit of muscle power.

Strong muscles help us center our bodies where needed and help us move where we want to when we have to, without us falling all over the place. Thus, muscles mean balance.

There are three ways of doing resistance training and you can try and then choose which one works best for you.

Some people go straight for the weights (barbells, dumbbells, and all the bells). However, if you've never touched a weight in your life, or at least haven't in years, make sure to start with lighter weights and gradually work yourself up to heftier options. Don't overdo yourself, it won't make you progress faster, only increase your chances of injury.

You could always try resistance bands. If you don't know what they are, they're these stretchy bands that come in different resistances (strengths). The same goes for them though, start light and add on the lbs as you grow stronger.

And lastly, if you feel that at the start, you're a bit too weak to handle any weights or resistance bands, start off simply by using your own body weight. It still works great while you get yourself strengthened up.

So, to get in some resistance training, you can:

- Lift weights.
- Grip a tennis ball.
- Exercise with resistance bands.

- Carry things (like groceries).
- Do specific exercises, such as overhead arm curls, push-ups, pull-ups, arm curls, etc.

For resistance training, do them for all of your major muscle groups at least twice a week. However, you don't want to exercise the same muscle group on any two days in a row. Go about it like this: for example, work out your arms on Monday, and then your chest on Tuesday, legs Thursday, and then your abdominal the next day, etc.

Balance

We've established that balance helps us not to fall over. Falling becomes very common and much more frequent as we grow older, which could mean we have a couple of broken bones and bruises waiting for pickup!

For this one, you can practice your balance by standing on one foot for a few minutes, walking heel to toe, or doing the "balance walk" a couple of times, standing up from a seated position with a focus on not wiggling around. A lot of lower body strength exercises will also help with your balance as you're working towards strengthening your leg and hip muscles. Then there are also some classes you can consider attending such as Tai Chi, Yoga, or Pilates. Do a minimum of four balance exercises three to six times per week, and you'll see that you're more on your feet in no time.

Flexibility

Stretching is key to improving your flexibility. Flexibility is much more than just being able to do the splits. It can help you do very ordinary things, such as looking over your shoulder to back out of your driveway, or tying your shoes in the morning. You could stretch in the morning when you wake up, before you go to bed, and most definitely before and after workouts to warm-up and cool-down muscles and avoid hurting yourself. Yoga, Pilates, and certain sports and exercises can also help with your flexibility.

In this chapter, if you haven't noticed by now, I won't go into so much detail about how all the different exercises benefit particular body parts and overall health. It will not only take forever but as said, being active in your lifestyle holds the same benefits as drinking water and having good nutrition. Always stretch before and after a workout. However, while focusing on flexibility exercises alone, do them two to three times a week.

Better Safe Than Sorry

Remember when those "cool kids" told you, you looked dumb walking around all geared up in a helmet, kneepads, and reflector jacket? I do, and you know what? Turns out I was my own cool kid all along because safety isn't lame, safety is smart.

- Always warm-up before exercises and cool-down afterward.
- Listen to your body (if you feel you're experiencing pain, slow down on things, or go see a doctor for some advice and recommendations).
- Drink plenty of water to support your endurance, while making sure to keep your electrolytes up.
- If you plan on exercising outside, like going for a jog in the park, make sure that you're aware of your surroundings.
- Layer things up! You can always take off some clothes if you feel you're getting too warm and then add on some more when the weather cools down again.

- Use the appropriate safety equipment and precautions to protect yourself from any injuries, such as wearing a helmet while out biking or having someone stand by you while you're lifting heavier weights.
- Don't hold your breath while you're doing strength exercises. It will only make things harder on yourself. Take a breath out when you lift or push weights, and breathe in when you soften.
- Consult a doctor if you're unsure whether or not you're allowed to do an exercise. Like when you're on certain medications, if you're at an unhealthy weight, have bad bones, or any other reasons you might have concerns.

ACTIVE HABITS

Once you've embraced exercise as a habit, you'll start to notice how much easier hitting the gym and making overall healthier choices will become.

As you know, a habit comes without thought, and imagine how great it would be to break a sweat without dreading or thinking about doing so? Well, you won't bust out in jogs while you're at a family dinner, but you'll have a healthier mindset to guide you through your new lifestyle.

Make sure that the exercise routine is suitable and convenient to your schedule. Once again, you don't have to turn and toss your schedule around, you can still set these habits in your life while your normal routine is intact.

To begin with, you could add some small workouts and exercises to things that are already a part of your life, such as dancing while you clean the house, or doing some exercises while seated at your desk.

Also, think about the time of day that's most comfortable and open for you. This could be the temperature, how busy you are at certain times of the day, how sore your muscles feel, and even the periods when you eat. There are a lot of things that could affect how you feel while exercising, as well as your motivation to begin in the first place. This could take a couple of days to weeks to get a precise grip on, but once you have it, you have it, and then you'll be able to scribble the rest of your exercise plan to fit around that.

On that note, another important throw-in to remember is to always be bendy. I don't mean you should split, twirl, and curl all day long. By being limber, I mean that you should always prepare for the unexpected.

Things that we don't want or think about often come around when we need them the least. Sadly, that's how it is and it's out of our control. You could, for example, get injured or have an important deadline at work that takes up all your time. This doesn't mean you have to stop old turkey or give up altogether. You could either still stick to small exercises (that don't involve your injured limb), or you can get back on track as soon as you're feeling better or have the time. Just adjust your workout habits to fit the change until everything is back to normal.

While we're on the topic of injury, also remember that the whole thing about "no pain, no gain," isn't what you think. Sure, when you start exercising (or increase the intensity of a workout), your muscles will be a bit sore and taut. That's completely normal, but there are countless tips and tricks there to fix that right up. However, if you experience any sort of pain or feel as though you might have injured yourself, call it a day and take a break.

Now, let's turn our focus to your routine itself. Firstly, remember that exercising doesn't have to be boring! There's nothing worse for me personally than exercising in dead silence and hearing my huffing-puffing all the way through! If you prefer that, that's you. Regardless, I prefer switching on some music, sometimes my favorite TV show while doing a quick aerobic burst.

You could do the exact same. Whether it's adding some spice to your exercise routine, or switching up the whole scene such as walking around the zoo instead of around the block.

Also, never stick to the same routine. A lot of people bore easily, and this could cause your motivation to plunge completely. Thus, mix things up every now and then. Go running as part of your aerobic routine one day, and then go row a boat or something the next.

Now, what you might have been waiting for all along: Here are some ways to make the ol' habit stick:

- Keeping Time: the best way to make sure you're always on time for your appointment with your exercise habit, is to set up some reminders. Such as alarms before your workout, calendar events so people know that you're unavailable at certain times, and then there's also an accountability system. You could tag along with a workout buddy or join a club or community center, which will hold you accountable if you weren't on time or chose to skip leg-day.
- Trackers and Co.
- Keep track of the exercises you've done throughout the day (you can also add the duration) to stay motivated. You'll see the list and realize, "Wow! I really can do this after all!" You could also keep an additional hard copy of the list. This way, you could scratch out the exercises as you complete them. I've found that it's kind of a trick-motivation tactic where it feels as though some sort of weight is being pulled from your back. The poundage gets lighter and lighter as the items fall from the list, and your goal starts to feel as light as a feather, meaning you'll clear off your entire routine.
- Once again, you can track these habits in a journal or digital space. While I'm here, I would like to add that

since I've mentioned journaling for all the habits so far (and will most likely bring it up again), you could either have one large journal to keep all your habits in one place, or, if you prefer keeping them separate, you could also carry a bunch of smaller logbooks, or just go digital.
- While you're at it, write down all the habits that you've coupled with exercising as a habit and all the goals you want to achieve. Put it down on a piece of paper, poster, or post-it notes. Then, smack it onto somewhere where you can see them both all the time, like near your mirror, so that you're always reminded of what you'll gain and where you're headed.

TAKE IT FROM JEFF

If you talk to Highschool Jeff, you would see that he was never the one to get involved in sports or any other physical activity for that matter. So, of course, the old school friends he bumped into at the shopping mall were surprised when they saw him dressed up in a neon gym vest and running shorts. "Training for a marathon," he told them, and that was his goal.

A few months back, Jeff decided that something in his life had to change. He had gained a lot of weight, so much so that he could barely pull on his socks. He was tired all the time, and when he wasn't tired, he got sick. What really bothered him was that he was no longer able to play with his son outside without gasping for air within a few seconds of briskly strolling outside.

Everything was spiraling out of control and had been that way for a while, so he made a plan. Jeff started by creating a healthy balanced meal plan, coupled with an exercise routine. He followed both of them sacredly. He noted that his immune system was picking up over time, as well as his performance when going for a jog, which he could credit to the great amount of water he consumed, and the amount of sleep he was getting as it got easier to breathe.

At first, Jeff wasn't training, that was until a charity marathon walked—or, jogged—into their city. He signed up right away, along with Mark, a friend from work. From there, both of them meet up early in the morning to go for a run, talking about business and their families to keep things interesting. After their run, they each head home and jump into the shower to unwind before they take their bicycles to work. No one recognizes Highschool Jeff anymore, and he's much happier being able to do the things he loves rather than hiding away.

DAILY DOSE OF IRON

This is a simple sample of an exercise routine for a single week, with 150-minute aerobic, arm-focused strength exercises, as well as balance and flexibility activities. Although, I'm not telling you to follow this exercise regime immediately once you start exercising; we all have different resources and body limitations. This is simply a program set up with the inspiration of a beginner's plan from Healthline (Semeco, 2021):

SAMPLE OF EXERCISE PROGRAM	
MON: 45-min moderate-pace jog or brisk walk.	**TUE:** 30-sec single-leg balance (each leg), 30-sec weight-shift (each side), 1-min walking heel to toe.
WED: 30-min brisk walk. Circuit #1: 8–12 lateral raises, 5–10 wall push-ups, 8–12 tricep dips. (*2–3 Sets*).	**THU:** Standing quad stretch, standing side stretch, shoulder stretch. *Hold every stretch for a count of 5 seconds.*
FRI: 30-min bike ride, hike, or moderate-pace jog. Circuit #2: 10 alternating chair-dips, 10 jumping jacks, and 10 squats (*2–3 Sets*).	**SAT:** Balance walk (*2–3 times*). Stretch from head to toe, holding stretches for 5–10 sec each.
SUN: 45-min run, jog, or take a long walk.	

Here's your activity:

- Sit down and create a one-week beginners plan of your own. Remember to make it personal and to keep in mind all of the factors in your life, such as what time you will start exercising, your current fitness level, resources, energy, temperature, etc.

Furthermore, here are some more things you could do. So, enjoy!

- Create a motivational board consisting of what drives you to change. Is it your family? Do you want to join a marathon? A tournament? Or do you have a certain health disease you want to keep under control?
- Also, add the benefits you'll get from having exercise as a habit in your life.
- Think about your goals and add them to your board.
- Keep a week's worth of entry into your exercise routine when you start exercising. Note down how you felt before you exercised after you exercised, and how you felt after the entire week. Did you feel any pain or discomfort? Is there anything you wish or feel you could've changed?

8

TAKING A STEP BACK

My dear friend, clear your mind of can't.
–Samuel Johnson

Over here! I've found that this habit is a two-in-one kind of deal: One part self-care and two parts clearing the mind (in other ways). Both of these are focused on shifting your mind and health to a new level, where you'll always be on the top of your toes, game, or whatever you wish to be on top of! Let's just jump right in!

WHAT'S THE PRIORI-TEA

We've already walked quite the road together, haven't we? With that said, you probably know that I'm that parrot on the pirate's shoulder because I fear I keep on repeating myself. However, I think I might have found a loophole, and here it is (Glowiak, 2020):

Engaging in a self-care routine has been clinically proven to reduce or eliminate anxiety and depression, reduce stress, improve concentration, minimize frustration and anger, increase happiness, improve energy, and more. From a physical health perspective, self-care has been clinically proven to reduce heart disease, stroke, and cancer. Spiritually, it may help keep us in tune with our higher power as well as realize our meaning in life. (para 3)

Most of the time, our brains get clogged up with all the stress and whatever pain life brings our way. However, to bring balance back into the equation, we need to take care of ourselves and clear our minds so that we can be leveled and healthy. This is a problem I know many of you struggle with: Putting others to the side and placing yourself at the front in line.

There are various reasons why you might have put barriers to self-care, such as feeling guilty, not having the time, you don't know what to do, a lack of planning, etc. But that's why you're reading this book, to make these changes and finally pick up some self-care for yourself. Nonetheless, we'll work through this together, it's essential for your health after all.

The overall intent of self-care is described as, "the way a person prevents and controls diseases as well as preserves their overall well-being through the uniform act of taking care of various dimensions of their health and life," (Bottaro, 2022).

When someone says "self-care," I can't help but imagine a person sitting on a plush armchair, wrapped up in a robe, hair toweled up, thick green face mask, cucumber eyes, and a cup of tea steaming in one hand. Turns out, I'm not the only one who thinks that self-care is only achieved if you do a specific set of activities.

However, that's not the case, as self-care is a much more outstretched and all life aspects come into play, the World Health Organization (WHO), listed these dimensions:

- Hygiene (general and personal)
- Take a long bath, set up a beauty routine, cut your hair every month or so, do your nails, get a shave, etc.

- Pick up rubbish you see on the street, avoid littering yourself, clean your home, garden, etc.
- Nutrition (which is a simple habit)
- Make time for healthy eating and drinking habits.
- Other factors that might affect your health are smoking, drug use, and excessive drinking.
- Lifestyle factors (such as your exercise level and leisure activities)
- Staying active is a habit as you know, such as exercising daily.
- Going for your annual check-up at the doctor, taking vitamins and immune boosters, etc.
- Leisure activities can be anything you can enjoy doing, such as going to the arcade or watching a good movie.
- A focus on your intellectual aspect of life, such as reading this book, watching a documentary, expressing your creative side, and things like that.
- Environmental factors (such as your living conditions or social habits)
- This could be that you find your home too cluttered, or you want to redecorate your office space. Maybe your neighborhood isn't the safest or your house is cramped, and you want to move out.
- Social is when you spend time with your family and friends, or you volunteer at your local dog shelter, for example.
- For me, this would also include an occupational dimension—where you could, for example, learn a new trade, polish up your resume, and even open up your own business.
- Socioeconomic factors (such as a financial situation or cultural/spiritual beliefs)

- You can sweeten the financial situation you're in by saving money, investing, cutting back on unnecessary expenses, etc.
- As for cultural and spiritual beliefs, this could mean getting in touch with your culture and practicing their traditions, practicing your religions, or something completely different such as meditating or doing right by others.

When we're setting up a self-care routine to follow, it will be very helpful to take a look at these facets, as together they help make us whole, and generally give us higher levels of health.

When we don't take time to self-indulge, as I've said, our mental and physical health won't be all rainbows and daisies. We'll also most likely experience problems with sleeping, holding, and caring for relationships, and a drop in self-esteem, empathy, and compassion (Ali, 2019). In sum, your health will not be where it could be, and although the other habits will help, you won't feel as whole, healthy, and happy as you should.

CLEARING THE WAY

Personally, I view clearing the mind as part of a self-care routine (which is why they're stuck together in this chapter). However, clearing the mind is more focused on mental and emotional health alone. It's a very powerful way to dump all the clutter you have so you could focus on what's important to you in life. This will particularly be useful once you start implementing all the simple habits in your life. You'll be able to focus on what's important and why you want to implement these habits, thus keeping your motivation fed. You'll also be able to think clearly about the actions you take, the temptations that surround you, and everything from *a* to *b* that stands in your way and helps you move forward.

Ways to Clear Your Mind:

- Write it down: Take the time to sit quietly, see what thoughts and feelings come to mind, and write them down.
- Exercise: It often helps you blow off some steam, so by implementing the previous habit, you'll kill two birds with one stone (hopefully not literally!).
- Reflect: Take your time to review how you're spending your time, what's causing stress in your life, what you feel lacks in your life, etc. Reflect on your life and decisions, this could be in the form of simply sitting back and thinking things through to sitting down to meditate.
- Talk about it: Sometimes you just need someone to listen while we rant. So, why not go out with some friends, or have some coffee with a family member and tell them what's been going on in your life, ask for some advice, or just ask them to be your shoulder.
- Sleep it off: Sleep helps you relax, and by all the benefits you know of, it can help take off some of the pressure you're experiencing.
- Take a breather: Sometimes, all you need is to breathe. Sometimes, everything seems to happen all at once, and you just need to stop what you're doing, close your eyes, then inhale and exhale.

YOGA-NA DO IT

We don't all enjoy the same activities, therefore the first step would be to envision and detail your self-care activities. These activities should be things you truly enjoy (and not just something you found on the internet), so that even during those times when life gets hectic, you actually look forward to jumping into your routine.

You have to put your foot down and get to the bottom of what's been holding you back from looking after yourself. Use these roots and patterns to help you overcome the bad habit you have of not taking on more time for self-care. Ask yourself why you feel the way you do? What can you do to put an end to it? And really, just have a stern talk and push on for some tough love!

You should also make sure that your self-care routine is somewhere that it fits in with your schedule. As I keep saying, you don't have to overthrow your entire life to make these changes, life can go on as usual. I know it might seem as though you need to open a lot of time and space (where there is none), but with some time management and re-evaluation of your life, you'll see that they slide right in.

Setting SMART self-care goals can also help plenty, especially if you've never been one to practice self-care or haven't done so in a while. But, if you find yourself struggling, you can try using self-love and goal-setting planners to help guide you. Once again, you can ask a friend or professional to help hold you accountable and lend you some advice too.

Remember that this routine should become a habit in the end, so you'll have to be consistent when completing it, or else it will just become something you do every once in a while until it fades away again. It would also help if you discuss these goals with those in your life. For example, you can ask your partner to look after the kids for five minutes while you complete this routine, and then you'll be back on duty.

Again, and I won't even explain it, keep track of your self-care habits by using journals, apps, and stuff like that. You know the rhyme: It will help keep you on track, motivated, and on your game (not much of a poet, sorry.) Just take things slow, and learn to love taking care of yourself. It might feel uncomfortable and strange at first, but I promise you, your body and mind will thank you later!

BARKING RIGHTS

Now, before I confuse you all, the following includes some images of dog training. I know—you're not a dog. However, I do think it will help illustrate the power of the mind.

My dog went through something. Some sort of canine-mid-life crisis? I'm not too sure what it was, one day he loved and trusted me, and then the very next he didn't trust me at all. It was heartbreaking and I was determined to find a solution to make my pup comfortable and have him come join me on the couch, instead of eyeing me from the corner of the room. That's when I stumbled onto something called the Trust Technique by James French.

The technique essentially teaches you how to be one with yourself through meditation. I can't give too much away since this is a product, but it's basically all about focusing on your surroundings and calming your animal to feel comfortable and safe around you. Through this intense focus on your surroundings, your mind naturally clears itself. It really didn't take more than a couple of minutes and my dog was more comfortable around me. I did this every day, and soon we were back to being best buds! I also did this every time I had to put his harness on when he had to go for a bath, had to clip his nails, or even when I just wanted to watch a movie with him. I know it isn't a lot of explanation, but still, I hope you get the picture.

I've found that out of all of the techniques I've tried for meditation, this one was the easiest to master. It was beneficial for both me and my dog, showcasing the clear benefits that come from clearing one's mind. In this case, I won my dog's trust and learned a new method that I used up to this day for more complex issues in my life. As all the teachings suggest, meditation helps remove all the tension that's in your body and mind. This specific method might not be for you, but there are so many more methods for you to try out, from sitting around and focusing on your breath to some guided meditations, peace is key.

CALMING CHORES

1. List some self-care activities you are interested in and why you're interested in them. When do you plan on finishing up your routine, etc? If you can, plan out everything. Make sure to include enough activities for a week at least. As well as alternative activities, for when you, for example, don't have enough time to do an activity that takes up more time.
2. Take a piece of paper or two (and a pen/pencil) and go sit outside. Take a few minutes to look around you and observe your surroundings. Focus on as much detail as you can, such as everything you see around you (like the orange leaves and the ants running on the ground), everything you feel (from the sand to the wind and sun), everything you hear (a neighbor cutting his grass and a dove chirping on the roof), and then everything you smell (the musty pollen of a flower, to the scent of gasoline somewhere). Write down all of these observations, trying to describe them in as much detail as you can, focusing only on those things and your senses.

9

BREATHING 101

When in doubt, look up to the sky and take a deep breath.
–Anon

Before we discuss what proper breathing looks like and means to you, let's look at how our bodies actually breathe.

Imagine I just threw that sketch of chapter one (of our bodies) in front of you. Colored in purple in the middle of your chest are two circular lobes with dangling tree-like shapes in red and blue. Those are your lungs, bronchi, and bronchial tubes, on the ends of some of them, there are these (rather gross looking) grapes, called alveoli or air sacs. There will also be a pipe-looking shape in the middle of your chest called the trachea (windpipe). Moving down only a bit, you'll see a dome-shaped muscle (it would be right under your ribcage). This is your diaphragm. While we're on ribs, the layer of muscles between them (which would be another poster) is called the intercostal muscles. That's the basics of the respiratory system, excluding, of course, your mouth and nose. Now that we know all of the building blocks to breathing, how do they work together?

It starts when you breathe in or out—the diaphragm tightens and moves downward. This allows your lungs enough space to inflate, and allows the lungs to shrink as well. The intercostal muscles between the ribs allow your ribcage to move along. When your lungs expand, the air is sucked through your mouth or nose and down your windpipe. From there, the air bounces through the bronchial tubes into the air sacs before being washed into the bloodstream. Simultaneously, carbon dioxide treks from the bloodstream to the air sacs before exiting the body when you exhale. (Thanks to Elliot's physical therapy for making it easier for me to explain.) And this is how we breathe!

Whether or not all of us breathe correctly, is where the habit steps in. The fundamental of breathing correctly lies in great posture. A lot of us tend to slouch and bend our bodies, thus we don't allow our lungs to fill up to their full capacity. With good posture, the lungs fill up with no hindrance. As for the exhale, make sure you're blowing out all of the air (carbon dioxide) from your lungs. With just these two pointers, you'll notice that you have a lot more energy and breath.

Look, we need oxygen. Without it, our bodies won't work. You know how people always say to "get some fresh air," they say this so that your mind clears up and you gather your thoughts. But this is literally what happens, though! When you breathe correctly, you'll find that you have more mental clarity and less stress. It also helps with your sleeping habits, keeps you healthy, and improves the body's immune system. Oxygen and breathing are the creation of life. So, why not do it right?!

LUNG LESSONS

In the following section, we'll go through how you could breathe more efficiently while molding it into your life as a habit.

Stomach and Nose

We have mouth-breathers and nose-breathers. Both get the job done. However, nose-breathers out there have a slight advantage in that the mouth can't filter, warm, or humidify air the way our nostrils do. That's why the nose is better, but we still have the belly to think about. When we breathe with our stomach, our diaphragm is engaged, and it does most of the hard work from there. The technique is best used when feeling rested. There are some breathing exercises to help you achieve this, which you'll spot below.

Breathing Exercises

Breathing exercises are great ways to practice the way you breathe, while also strengthening your lungs. Lucky for you, there are various breathing exercises out there for you to look at and use in your life.

Belly Breathing

1. Relax your shoulders and lie down or sit back in a chair.
2. Place one hand on your chest and the other on your stomach.
3. Inhale through your nose for a two-second count.
4. Feel how the air moves to the abdomen and your stomach pushes out, you'll notice that your stomach moves more than your chest.
5. Exhale for two seconds through pursed lips while pressing your stomach down.
6. Repeat a few times.

Pursed Lips Breathing

1. Inhale through your nostrils (once again for a count of two).
2. Purse your lips, like the pouting-selfie trend is back.
3. While keeping your lips pursed, breathe out slowly. This should take at least twice as long as it did when inhaling.
4. Repeat a few times.

These two are great for working on breathing with your diaphragm and opening up your airways. However, as said, there are many more exercises out there. Here are a few to get you started:

- 4-7-8 breathing technique (an old friend)
- deep breathing
- rib stretch
- numbered breathing
- coordinated breathing
- alternate nostril breathing
- huff cough

Healthy Air Containers

Breathing is our last simple habit. I know, stating the obvious, but why do I bring this up? Well, because all the other habits, in some way or another, help improve the way we breathe (well, all of them help each other out in the end.) Some examples you'll spot below, and some are encouraged by good breathing, etc.

However, first, let's take a look at how you can keep your lungs healthy and prevent getting a bit short-breathed:

- Stop smoking (and avoid secondhand smoke) and any other environmental irritants, such as smoke from machines and cars.
- Eat foods rich in antioxidants.
- Exercise frequently.
- Improve the air quality indoors. You can use certain things to help you get cleaner air inside your home, such as air filters. Also, reduce pollutants such as mold, dust, and artificial fragrances. Instead, go for natural alternatives (the fragrances… not the mold and dust…).
- Get regular checkups with a doctor, and if you're at risk for lung cancer ask your doctor about screening options.
- Wash your hands regularly.

KEEP BREATHING

Now here we are, left with one question: How can you take what you've so far learned and turn it into a habit? I mean, we literally breathe all the time, so how are we supposed to keep track of whether or not we're breathing *well*? I know, it sounds like quite the confusing ball game.

However, it's all about staying focused. Of course, you won't be able to focus on how you're breathing the whole day, but try to check up on it now and then.

You could, for example, set alarm intervals where you check your breathing and posture. If they're well, you could simply carry on, and if not you can reposition and fix them right up before checking in again later.

Also, do breathing exercises and lung strengthening exercises daily, this will help your mind form this new way of breathing habitually, while you're also ensuring some proper working lungs. You can still keep track of exercises in a journal (won't go on again, I promise), by listing which exercises you did, how long you did them, and how they felt. It's all about training your brain to recognize and remember these patterns until it knows them on the tips of its (metaphorical) fingers.

ANOTHER ONE FROM MY LIBRARY

I was suffering from chronic sneezing. I know it might sound silly and made-up, but I can assure you, it was definitely no jokes or fun and games for me. I got very ill and I was feeling terrible every single day! When I got to my doctor, he did his inspection and came back with a reason for my chronic sneezing: "You're not breathing properly, Ms. Kate."

This annoyed me so much at first! I was up in arms because obviously, I'm not *breathing* properly Doctor! I haven't had the chance to because I can't stop sneezing!

Nonetheless, an apple a day keeps the doctor away, they say—and for me, the apple was following his advice. I did a couple of breathing exercises every day, focused on how I was breathing with a proper technique, and within a few days or maybe a week, I could do all of those without having to take breaks to blow my nose. Things were looking up.

Look, I'm a health coach, and I can't diagnose or treat illnesses, so yes, the doctor was 100% right, and I admit my ways were wrong. However, I will most definitely throw some of the blame on my sneezing and the fact that I was feeling out of sorts, so...

Anyhow, that's water under the bridge now. Things are much better with me, thanks to the ol' doc. and proper breathing. I was so impressed I even bought a 3-ball spirometer! Which is just a device that helps you do some respiratory training.

WHEEZY WORKS

Choose a breathing exercise of your choice, preferably one that's focused on nose-and-belly breathing (and then obviously do it). Jot down how it felt for you:

Did it feel as though you were breathing better?
Were there any physical changes? Did you have more energy, did your mood change, etc?
Were there perhaps any parts that felt really uncomfortable for you to perform?

Check back in a week after doing this exercise, answer the same questions, and note down below if you experienced any other changes with your breathing. *For example; I felt that my sleeping pattern (and my snoring according to my partner), greatly improved since I began these breathing exercises. It feels as though my airways are much more open... And so on, and so on.*

WEEK 2: Did it feel as though you were breathing better?

WEEK 2: Were there any physical changes? Did you have more energy, did your mood change, etc?

WEEK 2: Were there perhaps any parts that feel really uncomfortable for you to perform?

THE LAST WORDS

We've walked together for a good few chapters now, and I'm sad to see you go. However, I know you're more than capable of doing this and living your best life with all these tools to get these six simple habits under your grip.

It won't be easy. Then again, I never said it would be. The greatest and the last piece of advice I would have to give you is to keep pushing on even when you're down on the ground with your bad days—even when there's not even a glimpse of progress hinting your way.

Remember, one bad day isn't the end of the world, just get back on that horse. Also, nothing happens overnight. As author Zig Ziggler once said, "There is no elevator to success. You have to take the stairs," (n.d).

You just have to be tough, (and I know you are), believe in yourself, and you know what, stop pulling yourself down, your *numero uno*! So, start acting like it! You'll do more for others by making sure you're around for longer, all healthy, and happy.

You now know what healthy habits look like, how to throw away the bad, and how each and every simple habit works and

THE LAST WORDS

contributes to your health; I know the dangers that come from ignoring them, and how to stay motivated to make drinking water, eating right, sleeping well, staying active, caring for your mind, and taking a breath, stick around. So, here's your promised first aid kit! Stocked up and ready for you to use (although, don't actually hurt yourself). All that's missing is you, and we're good to go.

I believe in you, and we've only been talking through typed words! Well, I did most of the talking. The point is that there's no better time than now, and if you're reading this, you're already halfway there, so keep going! And please, don't hesitate to reach out to ask me any questions or if you need some help. Even when you just want to get me back for all my chit-chatting. My hearing is excellent and my shoulders, I've been told, are quite sturdy!

So, here we are, and what more is there to say when everything has been said and done?

Well, I think a fitting way to say our goodbyes would be to quote one man who had the most exemplary commitment to habits in his life. However, be warned, he did not say these words one after the other, I had to paraphrase and stuff a whole bunch of his quotes together because they were all too suitable to pass up. So, let's hear it from the late and great, Albert Einstein:

How many people are trapped in their everyday habits; part numb, part frightened, part indifferent? To have a better life we must keep choosing how we are living.[...] We cannot solve these problems with the same thinking we used when we created them.[...] You can never fail until you stop trying.
–Albert Einstein

Wow, those chips really made me thirsty... Better grab myself some of that H_2O!

REFERENCES

AeroGuard Flight Training Center. (n.d.). *Parts of an airplane and their function*. AeroGuard. https://www.flyaeroguard.com/learning-center/parts-of-an-airplane/

Ali, S. (2019, January 6). *Why your self-care isn't working*. Psychology Today. https://www.psychologytoday.com/us/blog/modern-mentality/201901/why-your-self-care-isn-t-working#:~:text=Neglecting%20personal%20care%20can%20cause

Amidor, T. (2021, January 12). *Does drinking cold water boost your metabolism?* Food Network. https://www.foodnetwork.com/healthyeats/healthy-tips/does-drinking-cold-water-boost-your-metabolism

Authentically Del. (2021, December 21). *70 Important goal ideas for the 7 areas of life*. Authentically Del. https://authenticallydel.com/goal-ideas-for-the-7-areas-of-life/

REFERENCES

Balagam, I. (2021, October 29). *These 8 sleep trackers will assure you get the beauty sleep you need.* Healthline. https://www.healthline.com/health/sleep/best-sleep-trackers#A-quick-look-at-the-best-sleep-trackers

Baluja, J. (2019). FAU | *Breaking bad - how to identify and break bad habits.* Fau.edu. https://www.fau.edu/thrive/students/thrive-thursdays/bad-habits/index.php

Bernstein, S. (2021, April 23). *How to make exercise a healthy habit.* WebMD. https://www.webmd.com/women/exercise-habits

Bottaro, A. (2022, January 4). *Self-care is a trendy buzzword, but what exactly is self-care?* Verywell Health. https://www.verywellhealth.com/self-care-definition-and-examples-5212781

Brown, L. (2022, February 8). *Changing your diet could add ten years to your life – new research.* The Conversation. https://theconversation.com/changing-your-diet-could-add-ten-years-to-your-life-new-research-176494#:~:text=Studies%20have%20also%20shown%20that

Cambridge Dictionary. (2019). *Deprived meaning in the Cambridge English Dictionary.* Cambridge.org. https://dictionary.cambridge.org/dictionary/english/deprived

Cecelia Health. (2020, December 9). *Understanding habits and why they are important to our health.* Cecelia Health. https://www.ceceliahealth.com/understanding-habits-and-why-they-are-important-to-our-health/#:~:text=Habits%20are%20essential%20to%20our

REFERENCES

Centers for Disease Control and Prevention. (2021, May 16). *Benefits of healthy eating.* Centers for Disease Control and Prevention; U.S. Department of Health & Human Services. https://www.cdc.gov/nutrition/resources-publications/benefits-of-healthy-eating.html

Clark, A. K. (2021, November 18). *10 Goal-setting exercises for an accomplished 2022.* GenTwenty. https://gentwenty.com/goal-setting-exercises/

Clear, J. (2018a). *Habits guide: How to build good habits and break bad ones.* James Clear. https://jamesclear.com/habits

Clear, J. (2018b, November 13). *The 5 triggers that make new habits stick.* James Clear. https://jamesclear.com/habit-triggers

Clear, J. (n.d.). *Atomic habits.* [Online Image]. In Short Quotes. https://shortquotes.cc/wp-content/uploads/2020/11/876c9e03b18b9dac90ceea3fa4d57eea.jpg

Cleveland Clinic. (2021, October 28). *How does sleep affect your health?* Cleveland Clinic. https://health.clevelandclinic.org/sleep-and-health/

Cotter, J. (2019, July 11). *How did people clean their teeth in the olden days?* The Conversation. https://theconversation.com/how-did-people-clean-their-teeth-in-the-olden-days-119588#:~:text=Ancient%20Chinese%20and%20Egyptian%20texts

De Sio, F. (2021a, February 3). *Understand goal-setting theory to make your goal happen.* Lifehack. https://www.lifehack.org/898490/goal-setting-theory

REFERENCES

De Sio, F. (2021b, July 28). *4 Effective goal-setting templates to help you set goals*. Lifehack. https://www.lifehack.org/909482/goal-setting-template

Duff, K. D. (2021, January 17). *Motivation is what gets you started. Habit is what keeps you going*. KDD Philanthropy. https://kddphilanthropy.com/motivation-is-what-gets-you-started-habit-is-what-keeps-you-going/#:~:text=Jim%20Ryun%20said%2C%20%E2%80%9CMotivation%20is

Duhigg, C. (2012, March 5). *Habits: How they form and how to break them*. NPR.org. https://www.npr.org/2012/03/05/147192599/habits-how-they-form-and-how-to-break-them#:~:text=Neuroscientists%20have%20traced%20our%20habit

Dusseau, D. [Denise]. (n.d). *Words of wisdom quotes* [Pinterest post]. Pinterest. Retrieved from https://za.pinterest.com/pin/284008320228371547/

Einstein, A. (n.d.). *Albert Einstein quotes* [Online Image]. In Addicted 2 success. https://addicted2success.com/wp-content/uploads/2017/09/Albert-Einstein-300x189.jpg

Elliot physical therapy. (2017, September 26). *The importance of proper breathing for your overall health* | Elliot. Elliott Physical Therapy. https://elliottphysicaltherapy.com/importance-proper-breathing-overall-health/#:~:text=Every%20system%20in%20the%20body

Fadnes, L. T., Økland, J.-M., Haaland, Ø. A., & Johansson, K. A. (2022). *Estimating impact of food choices on life expectancy: a modeling study*. PLOS Medicine, 19(2), e1003889. https://doi.org/10.1371/journal.pmed.1003889

REFERENCES

familydoctor org. (1996, January 1). *The exercise habit.* Familydoctor.org. https://familydoctor.org/the-exercise-habit/#:~:text=Start%20every%20workout%20with%20a

Ford, H. (2020, May 19). *6 Side effects of not drinking enough water.* Www.henryford.com. https://www.henryford.com/blog/2020/05/side-effects-of-not-drinking-water

French, J. (2010, October 10). *Introduction to the trust technique with James French.* Www.youtube.com. https://www.youtube.com/watch?v=PnV5IIRvUNk&ab_channel=JamesFrench

Freutel, N. (2022, December 21). *Best sleep apps of 2021.* Verywell Mind. https://www.verywellmind.com/best-sleep-apps-5114724

Gilbert, R. (2016, July 15). *10 Exercises to improve your flexibility.* HealthifyMe Blog. https://www.healthifyme.com/blog/10-exercises-improve-flexibility/

Gill, I. [Ishra]. (n.d) *HugeDomains.com* [Pinterest post]. Pinterest. Retrieved from https://za.pinterest.com/pin/Ad2t0UuTJi4fnoVr_oH-8FJUW7V3CxWM9V4_VotBwRj-TCXZNVRxTvI/

Glowiak, M. (2020, April 14). *What is self-care and why is it important for you?* Www.snhu.edu. https://www.snhu.edu/about-us/newsroom/health/what-is-self-care#:~:text=Engaging%20in%20a%20self%2Dcare

Greenidge-Horace, R. (2021, September 25). *Why are habits more important than inspiration?* - Solutions With Rush. Solutionswithrush.com. https://solutionswithrush.com/why-are-habits-more-important-than-inspiration/

REFERENCES

Haines, C. D. (2022, January 16). *Insomnia: When to seek medical care.* WebMD. https://www.webmd.com/sleep-disorders/insomnia-when-seek-medical-care

Harvard Health Publishing. (2020, March 25). *How much water should you drink? - Harvard Health.* Harvard Health; Harvard Health. https://www.health.harvard.edu/staying-healthy/how-much-water-should-you-drink

Harvard University. (2019). *Healthy eating plate.* The Nutrition Source. https://www.hsph.harvard.edu/nutritionsource/healthy-eating-plate/

Healthcare Associates of Texas. (2018, September 16). *7 Signs you're not drinking enough water - Healthcare Associates of Texas.* Healthcare Associates of Texas. https://healthcareassociates.com/7-signs-youre-not-drinking-enough-water/

Healthline. (2018, July 25). *The 9 most important vitamins for eye health.* Healthline. https://www.healthline.com/nutrition/eye-vitamins#TOC_TITLE_HDR_9

Ho, L. (2020a, January 20). *What are goals? Achieve more by changing your perspectives.* Lifehack. https://www.lifehack.org/863723/what-are-goals#what-are-goals

Ho, L. (2020b, April 29). *A complete guide to goal setting for personal success.* lifehack. https://www.lifehack.org/874351/goal-setting#why-is-goal-setting-important

How to Track Your Sleep without Watch? *5 Sleep tracker apps without watch.* (2021, October 21). ShutEye. https://www.shuteye.ai/track-sleep-without-watch/

REFERENCES

Johns Hopkins Medicine. (2019). *The science of sleep: Understanding what happens when you sleep*. Johns Hopkins Medicine Health Library. https://www.hopkinsmedicine.org/health/wellness-and-prevention/the-science-of-sleep-understanding-what-happens-when-you-sleep

Krans, B. (2020, June 4). *Balanced diet: What is it and how to achieve it*. Healthline. https://www.healthline.com/health/balanced-diet#what-is-it

Leaders Edge. (n.d.). *The importance of habits*. Leader's edge. Retrieved May 11, 2022, from https://www.theleadersedge.org/blog/the-importance-of-habits

LeBlance associates. (2014, September 15). *Oral hygiene for kids*. LeBlanc & Associates Dentistry for Children. https://kidsmilekc.com/why-is-nutrition-important-to-oral-health/

Liles, M. (2021, January 10). *10 Free printable goal-setting worksheets that'll help you achieve anything*. Parade: Entertainment, Recipes, Health, Life, Holidays. https://parade.com/993372/marynliles/goal-setting-worksheet/

London, J. (2019, February 28). *Using a food journal can help you lose weight — and actually keep it off*. Good Housekeeping. https://www.goodhousekeeping.com/health/diet-nutrition/a26538542/food-journal/

Mana medical associates. (2016, July 22). *Develop healthy eating habits*. Medical Associates of Northwest Arkansas. https://www.mana.md/develop-healthy-eating-habits/

REFERENCES

Mayo Clinic. (2017). *Bronchioles and alveoli in the lungs*. Mayo Clinic. https://www.mayoclinic.org/diseases-conditions/bronchiolitis/multimedia/bronchioles-and-alveoli/img-20008702

Mayo Clinic Staff. (2020a, August 4). *Balance exercises: Step-by-step guide*. Mayo Clinic. https://www.mayoclinic.org/healthy-lifestyle/fitness/multimedia/balance-exercises/sls-20076853?s=2

Mayo Clinic Staff. (2020b, October 14). *Water: How much should you drink every day?* Mayo Clinic. https://www.mayoclinic.org/healthy-lifestyle/nutrition-and-healthy-eating/in-depth/water/art-20044256#:~:text=So%20how%20much%20fluid%20does

Mayo Clinic Staff. (2021, October 8). *7 Great reasons why exercise matters*. Mayo Clinic; Mayo Clinic. https://www.mayoclinic.org/healthy-lifestyle/fitness/in-depth/exercise/art-20048389

Migala, J. (2018, August 29). *The importance of healthy eating habits*. EverydayHealth.com. https://www.everydayhealth.com/diet-nutrition/importance-healthy-eating-habits/

Mitrokostas, S. (2021, April 23). *8 Signs you're drinking too much water*. Insider. https://www.insider.com/am-i-drinking-too-much-water-2018-11#:~:text=According%20to%20the%20MSD%20Manual

Motivation Supply. [Motivation Supply]. (n.d) *HugeDomains.com* [Pinterest post]. Pinterest. Retrieved from https://za.pinterest.com/pin/542120873873886165/

National Cancer Institute. (2019). *NCI dictionary of cancer terms*. National Cancer Institute; Cancer.gov. https://www.cancer.gov/publications/dictionaries/cancer-terms/def/alveoli

REFERENCES

National Institute of Diabetes and Digestive and Kidney Diseases. (2020, January 11). *Your digestive system & how it works | NIDDK.* National Institute of Diabetes and Digestive and Kidney Diseases. https://www.niddk.nih.gov/health-information/digestive-diseases/digestive-system-how-it-works#whathappens

National Institute on Aging. (2021, January 29). *Four types of exercise can improve your health and physical ability.* National Institute on Aging. https://www.nia.nih.gov/health/four-types-exercise-can-improve-your-health-and-physical-ability#endurance

Nunez, K., & Lamoreux, K. (2020, July 20). *Why do we sleep?* Healthline. https://www.healthline.com/health/why-do-we-sleep#:~:text=Many%20biological%20processes%20happen%20during

Onplanners.com. (n.d.). *Personal goal setting templates.* Onplanners.com. https://onplanners.com/templates/personal-goal-setting

Ortiz, K. G. (2013, March 28). *Quote by Kenneth G. Ortiz: "Be wary of the company you keep for they are...".* Goodreads. https://www.goodreads.com/quotes/767237-be-wary-of-the-company-you-keep-for-they-are

Otsuka Pharmaceutical Co. (n.d.-a). *Activities to convey the importance of rehydration.* Otsuka Pharmaceutical Co., Ltd. Retrieved May 11, 2022, from https://www.otsuka.co.jp/en/nutraceutical/about/rehydration/activities/

Otsuka Pharmaceutical Co. (n.d.-b). *The human body and water.* Otsuka Pharmaceutical Co., Ltd. https://www.otsuka.co.jp/en/nutraceutical/about/rehydration/water/body-fluid/#:~:text=The%20water%20we%20drink%20is

REFERENCES

Pai, A. (n.d.). *Water's journey through the body*. Aquasana.com. Retrieved May 11, 2022, from https://www.aquasana.com/info/waters-journey-through-the-body-pd.html#:~:text=Drinking%20filtered%20water%20is%20one

Queensland Health. (2018). *7 Amazing things that happen to your body while you sleep*. Qld.gov.au. https://www.health.qld.gov.au/news-events/news/7-amazing-things-that-happen-to-your-body-while-you-sleep

Quote Investigator. (2021, August 7). *You never fail until you stop trying – Quote Investigator*. Quote Investigator. https://quoteinvestigator.com/2021/08/07/never-fail/#:~:text=Albert%20Einstein%20said%2C%20%E2%80%9CYou%20never

Raymond, N. (2020, May 21). *Bruce lee's "be like water" quote explained*. ScreenRant. https://screenrant.com/bruce-lee-be-like-water-quote-meaning-explained/#:~:text=The%20Meaning%20Of%20Bruce%20Lee

Reiland, L. (2021, July 12). *Tips for drinking more water*. Mayo Clinic Health System. https://www.mayoclinichealthsystem.org/hometown-health/speaking-of-health/tips-for-drinking-more-water

Reliance Digital. (n.d.). *Water drinking habits and practices you must follow | | Resource Centre by Reliance Digital*. Www.reliancedigital.in. Retrieved May 11, 2022, from https://www.reliancedigital.in/solutionbox/water-drinking-habits-and-practices-you-must-follow/#:~:text=Making%20a%20habit%20of%20starting

Runner's World. (2011, May 23). *6 Ways to develop healthy eating habits*. ACTIVE.com. https://www.active.com/nutrition/articles/6-ways-to-develop-healthy-eating-habits

REFERENCES

Scott, S. (2017, July 10). *4 Free smart goal setting worksheets and templates*. Develop Good Habits. https://www.developgoodhabits.com/goal-setting-worksheet/

Selfcare Seeker. (2020, June 30). *13 Ways to find motivation for self care when it feels like too much work*. Self Care Seeker. https://selfcareseeker.com/motivation-for-self-care/

Semeco, A. (2017, March 2). *How to start exercising: A beginner's guide to working out*. Healthline. https://www.healthline.com/nutrition/how-to-start-exercising

Semeco, A. (2020, August 10). *20 simple ways to fall asleep fast*. Healthline. https://www.healthline.com/nutrition/ways-to-fall-asleep#2.-Use-the-4-7-8-breathing-method

Sequeira, A. H., Malik, R., Pandey, P., Chandra, R., & Baishya, P. (2014, February 8). *Study on drinking water habits of residents of a campus: A case study*. Papers.ssrn.com. https://papers.ssrn.com/sol3/papers.cfm?abstract_id=2392765

Shannon James Success Coaching. (2017, March 28). *Clear your mind to focus on what's most important*. Shannon James Coaching. https://shannonjamescoaching.com/clear-your-mind/#:~:text=Clearing%20our%20mental%20and%20emotional

Shoemaker, S. (2020, August 19). *12 Simple ways to drink more water*. Healthline. https://www.healthline.com/nutrition/how-to-drink-more-water

REFERENCES

SLE Education. (n.d.). My Sleep Reflection | *The importance of sleep | PDF Worksheet | PSHE | Teaching Resources.* Www.tes.com. Retrieved May 7, 2022, from https://www.tes.com/teaching-resource/my-sleep-reflection-the-importance-of-sleep-pdf-worksheet-pshe-12523396

Sparks, C. (2021a, May 25). *Behavior — Making your habits easier.* Medium. https://medium.com/@ForcingFunction/behavior-making-your-habits-easier-38d09eb4ee15

Sparks, C. (2021b, May 25). Triggers — *The key to building and breaking habits.* Medium. https://medium.com/@ForcingFunction/triggers-the-key-to-building-and-breaking-habits-fa8ed153ab0c

Sparks, C. (2021c, May 25). *Why habits are more important than we can imagine.* Medium. https://medium.com/@ForcingFunction/why-habits-are-more-important-than-we-can-imagine-d44628036117

Story, C. M. (2017, February 23). *Chronic lung diseases: Causes and risk factors.* Healthline. https://www.healthline.com/health/understanding-idiopathic-pulmonary-fibrosis/chronic-lung-diseases-causes-and-risk-factors#Lung-cancer

Suni, E. (2020, October 30). *What happens when you sleep: The science of sleep.* Sleep Foundation. https://www.sleepfoundation.org/how-sleep-works/what-happens-when-you-sleep

Suni, E. (2022, March 18). *Sleep deprivation: Causes, symptoms, & treatment.* Sleep Foundation. https://www.sleepfoundation.org/sleep-deprivation#:~:text=The%20term%20sleep%20deprivation%20refers

REFERENCES

The Berkey. (2020, January 14). *The Berkey*. The Berkey. https://theberkey.com/blogs/water-filter/where-does-water-go-after-drinking-it-the-explanation-of-water-absorption-into-the-body

The habit loop | Habitica wiki | Fandom. (2014, February 22). In Habitica Wiki. https://habitica.fandom.com/wiki/The_Habit_Loop#The_Reward

The USGS Water Science School. (2019, May 22). *The water in you: Water and the human body | U.S. Geological Survey*. Www.usgs.gov. https://www.usgs.gov/special-topics/water-science-school/science/water-you-water-and-human-body#:~:text=In%20adult%20men%2C%20about%2060

Troy, D. (2022, August). *Healthy sleep habits*. Sleep Education. https://sleepeducation.org/healthy-sleep/healthy-sleep-habits/#:~:text=Follow%20these%20tips%20to%20establish

True Fitness. (2021, August 12). *10 Simple arm-strengthening exercises*. True Fitness - Residential. https://shop.truefitness.com/resources/10-simple-arm-strengthening-exercises/

Walesh, S. (n.d.). *Using the power of habits to work smarter*. Www.helpingyouengineeryourfuture.com. Retrieved April 19, 2022, from http://www.helpingyouengineeryourfuture.com/habits-work-smarter.htm#:~:text=How%20much%20of%20what%20we

Watson, K. (2021, January 27). *Urine color chart: What's normal and when to see a doctor*. Healthline. https://www.healthline.com/health/urine-color-chart#colors

REFERENCES

Wax, D. (2008, July 7). *The science of setting goals (and how it affects your brain)*. Lifehack; Lifehack. https://www.lifehack.org/articles/featured/the-science-of-setting-goals.html

WebMD. (2020, August 10). *Slideshow: A visual guide to sleep disorders* (N. Ambardekar, Ed.). WebMD. https://www.webmd.com/sleep-disorders/ss/slideshow-sleep-disorders-overview

WebMD. (2021, April 14). *What happens to your body when you drink enough water?* (C. DerSarkissian, Ed.). WebMD. https://www.webmd.com/a-to-z-guides/ss/slideshow-drink-enough-water#:~:text=Water%20makes%20up%20a%20large

WebMD Medical Reference. (2020, August 24). *How much sleep do I need?* WebMD. https://www.webmd.com/sleep-disorders/sleep-requirements#:~:text=Most%20adults%20need%207%20to

West, M. (n.d.). *5 Reasons why it's important to develop good habits*. Thriveglobal.com. https://thriveglobal.com/stories/5-reasons-why-its-important-to-develop-good-habits/

Zephyr Cycling Studio. (n.d.). *The importance of habits: 5 Ways to actually stick with them* - Zephyr Cycling Studio. Zephyr Cycling Studio. https://zephyrcyclingstudio.com/2019/01/18/the-importance-of-habits/

Ziglar, Z. (2014). *Facebook post by Zig Ziglar* [Online Image]. In AZ Quotes. https://www.azquotes.com/quote/576536

ABOUT THE AUTHOR

Kate Tarratt Cross has made it her mission to inspire daily habits for healthy living which is why she became a health coach and author. Her varied and colorful life offered a host of diverse and unusual experiences but throughout her journey her underlying desire was to harness health and happiness which lead her to where she is today.

When she was just 20, she went to live in Haiti where she set up and ran an Art Centre for several years. While art was her first love, health was a close second. After obtaining her Art Degree in the UK she wanted to share what she had learned. The same can be said with the health and nutritional experience she's acquired.

After completing several art projects in both Haiti and her home country, South Africa, Kate had a vision to be surrounded by the color blue. She jumped on a sailing boat as a crew member and this is where she learned to cook and nourish others. She later became the private chef to many highly successful individuals.

From her experience as a creative, private chef and health coach and in particular from working in the personal environments of opulent and positive beings, Kate has accrued a wealth of insight into the importance of practicing good habits. It has been an ambition to write a book to serve those wanting to make positive changes and it is from her own adversity and life experience that she draws the inspiration to follow simple daily habits that can majorly improve our well-being and ultimately our happiness.

For more information visit Kate's website www.gowiththeglow.com.

Printed in Great Britain
by Amazon